For health care executives who are just
complex contracting process and for the
enced who require the most current info
the topic, *Managed Care Contracting* pr(
knowledge and tools they need to succeed.

G37
1999

THE AUTHORS

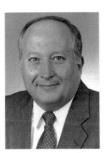

William A. Garofalo is
vice president of Health Care
Services with ML Strategies. He
is the former leader of health
care consulting for KPMG Peat
Marwick's New England region
and has worked nationally on a
variety of managed care projects.

Eve T. Horwitz is of
counsel with the Health Services
Group of the Mintz, Levin, Cohn,
Ferris, Glovsky, and Popeo law
firm. She routinely advises
physicians on managed care
issues as a member of the
American Medical Association's
Doctors' Advisory Network™.

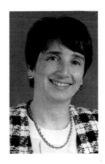

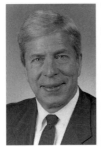

Thomas M. Reardon is
co-chair of the Health Services
Group of the law firm Mintz, Levin,
Cohn, Ferris, Glovsky, and Popeo.
He is a member of the board of
directors of Harvard Medical
Center and CRICO (professional
liability insurer for Harvard
affiliated teaching hospitals).

MANAGED CARE CONTRACTING

MANAGED CARE CONTRACTING

A Practical Guide for Health Care Executives

William A. Garofalo
Eve T. Horwitz
Thomas M. Reardon

Foreword by
Norman C. Payson, M.D.

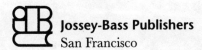
Jossey-Bass Publishers
San Francisco

Jossey-Bass books and products are available through most bookstores. To contact Jossey-Bass
directly, call (888) 378–2537, fax to (800) 605–2665, or visit our website at www.josseybass.com.

Substantial discounts on bulk quantities of Jossey-Bass books are available to corporations,
professional associations, and other organizations. For details and discount information,
contact the special sales department at Jossey-Bass.

 Manufactured in the United States of America on Lyons Falls Turin Book. This paper is acid-free
and 100 percent totally chlorine-free.

Library of Congress Cataloging-in-Publication Data

Garofalo, William A.
    Managed care contracting : a practical guide for health care executives / William A. Garofalo,
Eve T. Horwitz, Thomas M. Reardon.
        p.   cm
    Includes index.
    ISBN 0-7879-4581-1 (pb : alk. paper)
    1. Managed care plans (Medical care)—United States. 2. Medical care—Contracting out—
United States. I. Horwitz, Eve T. II. Reardon, Thomas M. (Thomas Michael) III. Title.
    [DNLM: 1. Managed Care Programs—organization & administration—United States.
    2. Contract Services—organization & administration—United States. W 130 AA1 G237m 1999]
    RA413.5.U5G37   1999
    362.1'04258'0973—DC21
    DNLM/DLC
    for Library of Congress   98-43360

FIRST EDITION
HB Printing   10 9 8 7 6 5 4 3 2

CONTENTS

CONTENTS

FOREWORD

Norman C. Payson, M.D.
President and Chief Executive Officer, Oxford Health Plan

As the president and chief executive officer of a large managed care organization, I may view managed care contracting issues from a different vantage point than do some in the provider community, which is the intended audience for this publication. However, I offer one business principle that is true from either side of the issues involved in managed care contracting: an informed and knowledgeable "participant" is always respected and appreciated. Bringing these characteristics to both sides of the negotiating table leads to a more expeditious and balanced negotiating process—a solid foundation for a business relationship.

On a personal note, I have had the opportunity to work with the authors on a variety of occasions. While I was president and CEO of Healthsource, Inc., I worked closely with Eve Horwitz and Tom Reardon on several issues, including Healthsource's acquisition of a not-for-profit HMO in Massachusetts. Their counsel was critical in successfully executing an extremely complicated transaction. For his part, Bill Garofalo was instrumental in assisting Healthsource in establishing operations in several states, including Arkansas and Ohio. Interestingly enough, in both instances Bill was representing the interests of providers, but his insight and direction led to a joint-venture arrangement that was mutually beneficial. His organized but sensitive approach to the process was pivotal to the agreements.

I hold the authors and their firms—ML Strategies, Inc. and Mintz, Levin, Cohn, Ferris, Glovsky and Popeo, P.C.—in the highest regard

PREFACE

Physicians (and most health care professionals, for that matter) have trained as scientists. Therefore, they are accustomed to making decisions based upon pertinent information. So, it's not surprising that when faced with standard managed care contracts, physicians want to do more than just sign on the dotted line. "Do more" usually means turning to the reimbursement schedule before deciding to sign. But the sections of the contract dealing with how the managed care organization administers its products and program, too often overlooked, are of equal importance.

Managed Care Contracting was developed to address the need that many of our physician and hospital clients have expressed for guidance in evaluating contracts and negotiating agreements. The book presents an overview of the issues involved in managed care contracting and offers practical ways for providers to prepare to operate in a managed care environment. Although it cannot replace the individual and specific advice physicians and hospitals should seek from attorneys and other expert consultants, it can help them take their place at the negotiating table across from managed care organizations with authority and confidence.

Payors come to the table with specific payment methodologies and contract provisions in mind. Providers who prepare in advance are in the best position to respond to opportunities to make a better contract, rapidly and effectively, and are more likely to benefit from entering into risk contracts.

We believe *Managed Care Contracting* addresses the contracting questions of physicians and hospitals alike. Interestingly, as more and more managed care contracting is integrated across provider lines, the objectives for physicians and hospitals become less distinct. More important, however, is the fact that physicians are the ultimate decision makers when it comes to patient care. To achieve the efficiency of operations required for success under capitation, physicians must understand the incentives and dynamics of capitation arrangements that directly affect them or the hospitals where they admit patients.

Chapter One outlines the steps an organization should take in entering into a risk-based contracting relationship with a managed care organization, including clarification of goals and objectives, assessment of operational strengths and weaknesses, and evaluation of the managed care plans. It also stresses the importance of identifying a negotiating team for your organization, first to include experienced legal and financial experts and second to involve in the negotiations individuals from operating areas within your own organization who can identify specific operational limitations or other contractual concerns.

Chapter Two provides guidance on developing a contracting strategy. Simply put, a contracting strategy involves tailoring your action plan into a strategy that matches your goals, objectives, and unique strengths to the needs of a specific managed care organization. Competitive facts that should be weighed are the provider's and the managed care plan's respective market shares, reputation, and leverage and the nature of the target market. Because your contracting strategy may involve responding to or issuing a request for a proposal, guidance on typical RFPs is provided in this chapter.

Chapter Three provides help in evaluating a proposal from a managed care organization, including its most critical components: the payment arrangement and the degree of risk for the provider. Understanding and evaluating the degree of risk is essential to tailoring a sound risk contract.

Chapter Four lays out the most important steps of a successful negotiation. The essential elements of negotiating a risk contract include understanding the payor's objectives and your own limitations, identifying all pertinent issues, performing a financial analysis, and preparing an executive notebook on each payor. Negotiating pointers are designed to help providers reach needed compromises with payors.

Chapters Five and Six present sample hospital and physician contracts. Additional commentary is provided to define key sections and direct attention to important issues.

Chapter Seven takes the provider to the step following negotiation of the contract, namely organizing managed care operations, which are often highly fragmented. It also provides recommendations for delineating key roles and responsibilities and using information systems to support managed care operations.

Chapter Eight offers concluding comments and final guidance. During the 1990s, health care underwent a sea of change in reimbursement and risk sharing. What is to come in the next ten years is anybody's guess. However, there is no doubting the continuing need for astute negotiations between providers and payors. What's more, there will be expanded opportunities for them to develop together creative approaches to contracting. Understanding the incentives and goals of providers and payors helps both parties and the health care community overall reach the optimum of quality, access, and cost-effectiveness in delivering health care services.

Acknowledgments

The authors would like to acknowledge and thank current and former members of the ML Strategies staff who contributed to researching, writing, editing, and preparing the final manuscript, especially Gail Allen, Carolyn Castel, Michelle Norman, and Susan Shea.

Boston, Massachusetts   William A. Garofalo
October 1998   Eve T. Horwitz
                                                         Thomas M. Reardon

THE AUTHORS

William A. Garofalo is vice president of health care services with ML Strategies, Inc., a consulting firm specializing in health care restructuring. Currently, he focuses his skills on major health care delivery system integration projects. These projects concentrate on a variety of corporate structures that align physicians, hospitals, and managed care companies in a coordinated manner with complementary incentives. This work entails strategic and business planning, physician education, information systems assessment, and financial modeling, as well as operational implementation.

Previously, Garofalo was the KPMG Peat Marwick partner responsible for health care services in the New England region. In addition to this regional responsibility, he was one of the firm's managed care leaders and oversaw most of its major engagements with health maintenance organizations and other managed care organizations. Prior to consulting, Garofalo was chief operating officer of a 450,000 member HMO and the executive director of a large multispecialty academic group practice at Johns Hopkins. This $100 million physician corporation managed three HMOs, fifteen health centers, a captive insurance company, and a proprietary fee-for-service billing company.

In the managed care area, Garofalo has been involved in HMO development, valuations and acquisitions, information systems definition and vendor selection and implementation, product planning, and operational reviews and mergers. He has also conducted a variety of provider network development and strategic-planning

studies. In regard to contracting, he has been involved in a variety of contracting negotiations with providers, insurers, outsourcing companies, and PBMs.
His physician-related activities have centered around group practice development,
HMO contracting, practice valuation and acquisition, developments in physician
hospital associations and independent practice associations, practice management
and physician billing, and clinical system selection and implementation.

Garofalo holds a B.A. in international economics from Rutgers College and
an M.B.A. in health care management from Boston University. He has lectured
nationally and internationally on a variety of business planning, physician, and
managed care topics.

Eve T. Horwitz is Of Counsel to the law firm of Mintz, Levin, Cohn, Ferris, Glovsky
and Popeo, P.C., and practices in its health law section. She also conducts an independent legal practice in Lexington, Massachusetts. Her practice involves all aspects of managed care, including advising HMOs, preferred provider
organizations, IPAs, and PHOs on corporate and strategic matters including planning and formation, contract negotiations, acquisitions, and regulatory compliance. She also routinely represents hospitals, nursing homes, durable medical
equipment manufacturers and suppliers, and other providers in their negotiations
with managed care entities and other third-party payors. Her practice also includes
representation of individual physicians, single and multispecialty group practices,
and other health care providers regarding corporate planning and formation; review of professional employment, services agreements, and management contracts;
and mergers, acquisitions, and sales of practices. Previously, Horwitz served as a
legal consultant to the federal Office of Health Maintenance Organizations.

Horwitz has been in the private practice of law for almost twenty years. In addition to her law degree, which she received from Boston University School of Law
in 1980, she has an M.B.A. in health care management from Boston University. She
received her A.B. from Mt. Holyoke College in 1976. She is on the American Medical Association's Doctors' Advisory Network™, is education coordinator of the Massachusetts Bar Association's Health Care Council, is a member of the American
Health Lawyers Association, and is a frequent lecturer at local and national seminars.

Thomas M. Reardon is president of ML Strategies, Inc., a former member of the
executive committee of the law firm of Mintz, Levin, Cohn, Ferris, Glovsky and
Popeo, P.C., and cochairman of the firm's health law section.

Reardon has served as a member of the board of Harvard Medical Center
and a member of the board and executive committee of CRICO (the offshore
professional liability insurer for Harvard University, the Harvard-affiliated teaching hospitals, and Massachusetts Institute of Technology). He currently serves as
a trustee of the Massachusetts Eye and Ear Infirmary, where he previously was

acting president from 1990 to 1992, and as chairman of the board through 1994. He is a corporation member of the Partners HealthCare System, the parent company of Massachusetts General Hospital and Brigham and Women's Hospital, and has served as a trustee of the American Trauma Society; he has also been a faculty member at the Harvard School of Public Health. Reardon serves as director for L. Gilbraith (the offshore professional liability insurer for a seven-hospital Midwestern health care system). He is on the investment advisory board of Hambro American Biosciences and has served as chairman of the business advisory board of a venture capital firm interested in early-stage funding of medical research; he has served as a director and officer of the National Commission on the Accreditation of Trauma Centers. He was chairman of the board of a large multispecialty medical group practice and is a columnist with *Hospital News*. More recently, he agreed to serve as a director on the boards of ZCI, a South Carolina-based occupational health and workers' compensation company, and Chapman Health International, Inc. He has served as a director of HealthAlliance, a multihospital health care system. He is a frequent lecturer and has published approximately one hundred articles on health care issues.

Reardon has been in the private practice of health law since his graduation from Harvard Law School in 1971. He has extensive responsibility for coordinating representation of major health care clients, including pharmaceutical companies, hospitals and hospital systems, multispecialty group practices, and managed care plans across the country. He possesses extensive experience in all aspects of health law and regularly advises health care organizations on strategic issues, including vertical and horizontal integration, strategic alliances, managed care and physician integration strategies, and market positioning.

With offices in Boston and Washington, D.C., ML Strategies is a unique multidisciplinary consulting firm specializing in health care services and biomedical products. ML Strategies helps organizations rethink their competitive positions; execute change; and coordinate the complex services needed for strategic, management, financial, legal, and communications planning and project implementation.

The *ML* of ML Strategies is the law firm of Mintz, Levin, Cohn, Ferris, Glovsky and Popeo, P.C., with more than 250 attorneys in offices in Boston and Washington. Mintz Levin is noted for its strengths in health care, corporate finance, technology, communications, real estate development, and litigation. Mintz Levin's health law section unites lawyers skilled in the different aspects of health law to address the diverse, complex challenges and opportunities encountered by clients in all segments of the health care industry.

Through its attention to the interplay between a client's legal issues and business goals, Mintz Levin and ML Strategies have built strong, long-standing professional relationships and developed an international network of business resources.

MANAGED CARE CONTRACTING

INTRODUCTION

As the future of health care is debated in America, a central question is whether medical care is not only a social good, but a right. If "health care for all" is determined to be a right, then who should bear the associated costs? Society as a whole? Employers? Or should individual employees pay the cost of their own medical care and medical care for their dependents? As yet, there is no definitive answer. Instead, the response has been a patchwork of private and public programs that provide health insurance for 85 percent of the population. Despite Americans' attempts to derive a truly workable system, the result has been "a paradox of excess and deprivation"[1]—and high cost.

Government spending for health care as a percentage of all federal expenditures was 12 percent in 1980 ($69 billion); by 1990 this figure had risen to 15 percent ($191.5 billion). Until recently, total health care expenditures were rising by approximately 12 percent every year. The growth of health care expenditures has now slowed, however, through rapid market development of managed care plans and because of the decision by many large employers to self-insure the health care needs of their own employees and their dependents. Many employers are also encouraging their employees to switch from traditional indemnity insurance to managed care plans, and some no longer offer traditional indemnity insurance coverage because premium increases have been too high.

In addition, many hospitals are willing to negotiate prices, and insurers are able to pay on a discounted per case or per diem basis. Third-party payors are also trying to make consumers increasingly sensitive to the financial implications of health care decisions by employing incentives such as lower insurance premiums to encourage use of lower-cost providers, alternative delivery sites, and shorter hospital stays.

In this environment, managed care organizations (MCOs), such as HMOs (health maintenance organizations), PPOs (preferred provider organizations), and IPAs (independent practice associations) have become increasingly popular with both payors and consumers. These organizations typically attempt to keep health insurance premiums below those of indemnity payors by restricting their provider networks to low-cost, efficient hospitals, physicians, and other service providers and by managing the care of their enrollees within their networks.

Managed Care Plans: Models and Selected Features

The rapid development of managed care plans is a reaction to escalation of health care costs over the rate of inflation and to the belief that managed care can produce demonstrable savings as compared to the costs associated with traditional fee-for-service indemnity health insurance. Managed care is generally seen as linking delivery of appropriate medical care to the financial aspects of health insurance.

Certain features are consistent across the variety of managed care plans:

- A selective network of contracted providers
- Enrollees who pay a predetermined monthly premium to the plan for covering a predefined set of health benefits
- A defined medical management program agreed to under contract with the network of providers
- Financial incentives and disincentives to help steer enrollees to selected providers
- Some degree of financial risk sharing with the network providers

The concept of managed care had its origins during the 1930s with such entities as the Health Insurance Plan of New York (HIP), Kaiser Permanente, and Group Health of Puget Sound. Groups of physicians served the enrollees, who all paid the same premium. Basically, the "passive" enrollees subsidized the "active" or sick enrollees. However, organized medicine strongly opposed these plans for decades, and they remained peripheral to the mainstream of American health care.

By the early 1970s, the Nixon administration determined that these prepaid group practices were a means of slowing down the ever-increasing cost of health care. By 1973, the Health Maintenance Organization Act was legislated. In the

1970s, the federal government spent hundreds of millions of dollars in developmental subsidies to increase the number of HMO plans. These actions alerted organized medicine to the fact that legislative action to reform the health care system was not beyond the realm of possibility. In reality, the government has not been as successful as the private sector in enrolling Medicare- and Medicaid-eligible beneficiaries. Efforts to migrate more of these beneficiaries into managed care have increased dramatically in the last few years.

The growth of private sector (commercial) HMOs did not accelerate until the 1980s. That accelerated growth was due to a variety of factors, among them increasing employer concern about health care costs; commercial carriers began to see that the health care indemnity insurance industry was in financial jeopardy, and traditional fee-for-service practitioners began associating with HMOs. From 1980 through 1995, enrollment in HMOs increased from 10.2 million to nearly 60 million.[2] Growth in PPOs was also dramatic.

Managed care plans are divided into three types, differentiated by the organization of physicians within the plans: staff model, group model, and IPA. In the staff model, physicians are salaried employees of the plan and treat plan enrollees in centralized treatment centers. In the group model, the plan contracts with physicians organized into group practices. Enrollees are treated in the private offices of the contracting physicians. The physician groups are reimbursed either according to an agreed-upon fee schedule or on a per member, per month basis (PMPM) under a capitation contract. The IPA model is the most common type of HMO, in which physicians contract to treat plan enrollees in their own offices. The physicians are reimbursed according to an agreed-upon fee schedule or on a PMPM basis under a capitation contract. Unlike those in the group model, IPA physicians are not organized into formal group practices.

The professional services contracts that physicians execute with managed care plans define the responsibility the physicians accept to provide comprehensive care for a fixed fee in exchange for autonomy in the practice of medicine; any oversight is carried out by peers, not external reviewers. In the group and staff models, the type and amount of care provided to enrollees is controlled by carefully developing a network of providers that matches enrollee health needs with the specialty and number of physicians in the plan's network. This network definition counterbalances the practice autonomy given to providers. Most often, specialty referrals are approved after the primary care physician, acting as a case manager or "gatekeeper," makes a referral. Through defining a selective network and requirements for authorization, the managed care plan maintains adequate access to primary care as well as productive patient schedules for its selected specialists.

In addition, many managed care plans incorporate financial incentives into their professional services contracts with physicians. Primary care physicians, and sometimes specialists, often share in financial surpluses generated as a result of underutilization of the medical services estimated to be required for an enrolled population. The debate regarding the appropriateness of such incentives or bonuses among health care consumers, advocates, and regulators is ongoing.

And Now, PPMCs and PSOs

California, Arizona, Minnesota, Massachusetts, Illinois, Ohio, and Florida are all considered to be states with "mature" managed care markets. Notwithstanding that these states have significant penetration of managed care, the degree of financial risk sharing between the managed care plans and providers varies widely. The highest degree of financial risk sharing is seen in California, Minnesota, and Florida, in which states the move to provider integration first gave birth to organized physician groups, such as physician hospital organizations (PHOs) and physician organizations (POs). The latest evolution is the physician practice management company (PPMC), acting as a conduit between insurer and provider.

PPMCs, many of which are publicly traded, fill the role of an IPA manager in negotiating managed care contracts on behalf of providers and applying proven medical management to the risk arrangements they negotiate in order to maximize the arbitrage from the capitation dollar. The success of PPMCs varies based upon their ability to garner national managed care contracts and to supply physicians and other providers with classic back-office services more cheaply and more efficiently than integrated providers can on their own.

In this same arena, providers have yet another option: provider-sponsored organizations, or PSOs. Providers weighing a decision to qualify as a PSO should consider the variety of standards they need to meet, including approval of all marketing materials by the federal Health Care Financing Administration (HCFA), payment rate changes, establishment of a coordinated grievance and appeals process, and additional comparative-data requirements.

On the positive side, PSOs are perceived to have the potential to improve care and lower costs, as well as other pluses:

- The care provided is anticipated to be more complete since providers follow their own medical management protocols, not those imposed by an insurance company or managed care plan.
- Care is more focused on community need, with care integrated—especially for the chronically ill—into the community based upon the needs and age of the population, available resources, and other factors. Further, access to care improves because providers in the PSO have direct referral protocols.

- PSOs may prove to have better technology and state-of-the-art information systems than older systems now in use.
- PSOs result in savings for the Medicare program because payment rates to PSOs are comparable to rates paid to managed care plans rather than the higher Medicare fee-for-service rates for the same services.
- PSOs are likely to increase competition as they offer another plan option for consumers and employers.
- PSOs are seen as a means of aligning providers more closely with patients because they are devoid of bonus structures and restrictions on medical management that may affect treatment decisions.

On the other hand, there are potential negative elements associated with PSOs, chiefly in the area of increased administrative responsibility:

- Besides delivering care, providers have to manage risk, build and maintain management infrastructure, and handle all of the back-office functions heretofore supplied by managed care plans or indemnity insurers.
- Many potential PSOs are building infrastructure from the ground up and do not have on hand professionals with experience in claims processing, member services, sales and marketing, provider services, and managed care financial management. Because PSOs, in effect, replace insurance company functions, they may employ third-party administrators (TPAs) to handle many management functions.
- Finally, PSOs may be viewed by consumers as an attempt on the part of providers to maximize earnings by cutting out the managed care organizations.

However PSOs are viewed, managed care contracting remains central to their success or failure.

A New Wrinkle: Patient's Bill of Rights

As the managed care industry continues to evolve and participation in managed care plans grows exponentially, contract negotiations are now facing a new challenge: the effect of state and federal legislation associated with "patient's rights."

State legislators throughout the United States are introducing dozens of bills in an attempt to govern how managed care plans operate. Concerned with maintaining a high standard of care in a time when cutting costs is a priority, advocates of these bills seek to guarantee certain rights for patients. They want to protect patients' autonomy to choose their health care providers and ensure that patients have access to treatments that are appropriate and necessary. In February 1998, President Clinton also jumped onto the bandwagon when he released an executive order prescribing that all federal health plans comply with the Quality Commission's Consumer Bill of Rights.

Although patient's bills of rights, or "patient protection acts," are often grouped under one general umbrella, many of these bills target specific issues: patient disclosure, direct access, emergency room services, and minimum lengths of stay. According to *Washington Health Week*,[3] as of 1997 twenty-four states had passed legislation pertaining to patient disclosure. These laws prohibiting so-called gag clauses have a direct effect on physician contracting. This type of legislation allows physicians to discuss any medically appropriate treatment, even if it requires patients to go outside of a managed care plan's network. The physician cannot be relegated to discussing only treatment options within the plan.

Twenty states have approved bills pertaining to emergency room services. This form of legislation ensures that if a "reasonably prudent" person feels that receiving emergency care is warranted, then the health plan should be responsible for covering that care. Another common patient rights law governs the minimum length of stay for certain procedures. Thus far, twenty-two states have passed laws governing minimum length of stay for delivery of a baby, and fourteen have approved minimum stay for mastectomy. Advocates for minimum stay after delivery assert that many of the common health-related problems that newborns encounter—such as dehydration, jaundice, and infection—are hard to notice in the hours immediately following birth. They argue that managing costs must not jeopardize the health and appropriate care of newborns.

Direct-access laws, which ensure that members of managed care plans have access to specialists without referral from their primary care provider, have been passed by fourteen states. Other laws that have been passed by legislators around the country include external grievance review (nine states), mental health parity (eight states), and "any willing provider" (seven states); eleven states have passed laws that restrict managed care plans from using financial incentives to influence the behavior of providers or enrollees.

These are merely a sampling of the diverse laws that are being advocated by health care watchdog groups, government officials, and plan members. With the landscape of both health care and managed care constantly changing, it is necessary to be aware of these legislative developments. Even more important, it is essential to keep these changes in mind when devising your strategy for contracting. From the provider perspective, the impact of these laws and the ability of the MCOs with which your organization contracts can affect the health care coverage your employees choose and receive, as well as the amount of the premium dollar allocated to plan management and out-of-plan medical services.

Risk contracting raises myriad issues for providers who are just beginning to deal with managed care organizations. *Managed Care Contracting* is designed to present an overview of the issues involved and to offer practical ways to prepare to operate in a managed care environment. It is intended to supplement—not supplant—advice rendered to a provider by its own attorneys and financial advisors.

Notes

1. Enthoven, A., and Kronick, R. "A Consumer-Choice Health Plan for the 1990s: Universal Health Insurance in a System Designed to Promote Quality and Economy." *New England Journal of Medicine,* Jan. 5, 1989, vol. 320, pp. 29–37.
2. Data from American Association of Health Plans (formerly known as Group Health Association of America).
3. "Blues Plans Expect States to Push Consumer Protections in 1997." *State Health Week,* Feb. 24, 1997, p. 2, supplement to *Washington Health Week,* Feb. 24, 1997, *5*(7).

CHAPTER ONE

PLANNING FOR MANAGED CARE RISK CONTRACTING

The steps an organization should take in entering into a risk-based contracting relationship with a managed care organization include:

1. Clarifying goals and objectives
2. Assessing operational strengths and weaknesses
3. Evaluating the managed care plans

It is important for an organization to identify a negotiating team that encompasses experienced legal and financial expertise, and to involve individuals from operating areas who can identify specific operational limitations or other contractual concerns.

Before considering entering into a risk-based contracting relationship with a managed care organization, health care providers are well advised to do some internal preplanning. A well-developed action plan provides the basis for all managed care contracting decisions. By developing such a plan, there is less chance of signing a contract that is at odds with your organization's goals or that is financially unprofitable. There is also less risk of exposure to unforeseen circumstances as a result of ambiguities in a contract.

The planning effort should include:

• Clarification of your goals and objectives

- Assessment of your operational strengths and weaknesses
- Evaluation of the managed care plans with which you might seek to contract

Identify Organizational Goals

The first step in developing a managed care contracting strategy is to decide how much risk, and what type, your organization is able and willing to bear. Willingness to assume risk may be related to your position in the market and your need to maintain or increase utilization. Additionally, it is important to understand the interests and motivations of all parties, including other providers (for example, hospitals, primary care physicians, specialty care physicians, skilled nursing facilities, home health agencies). The following list of potential organizational goals and questions may help you identify and prioritize your key objectives in the managed care marketplace.

Desire to Maintain Market Share

Have admissions or patient visits been declining? Are declines due to a decrease of population in your area? Or is a loss of patients due to shifts in enrollment from indemnity to managed care plans with which you do not currently contract? Are traditional indemnity programs considered too expensive by local employers?

Desire to Increase Market Share

Could an alliance make you an exclusive or preferred provider for specific unions or major employers? Has the local population been growing, thus potentially generating incremental volume if you increase your resources and outreach? Do you wish to increase your geographic base, and is there an opportunity to do so? Is there an opportunity to preempt other providers?

Desire to Change Composition of Patient Pool

Are you able to identify which services are most utilized and those that are underutilized? Has the DRG (diagnostic-related groups) payment adversely affected the profitability of high-volume diagnoses?

Desire to Decrease Your Days in Receivables

Are your accounts receivable long overdue? Have you had problems collecting from employed patients? Is your cost of collection, including lost revenue, greater than the discount requested?

Desire to Increase Nonoperating Revenue

Is the health care industry heavily regulated in your state? Is nonoperating revenue excluded from rate-setting revenue?

Desire to Attract or Maintain Medical Staff

Are physicians taking a leadership role in local managed care organizations? Are physicians who normally admit to your hospital participating in these plans? Is there an opportunity to influence admitting preferences?

Need to Play Follow the Leader

Have your competitors contracted with managed care organizations? Are colleagues from other geographic areas encouraging your participation in these plans?

Assess Organizational Strengths and Weaknesses

As a second step in preparing a contracting strategy, clearly identify the organization's perceived strengths in the market. These might include such factors as financial depth, reasonable cost structure, accessible locations, comprehensive service mix, good physician relationships, state-of-the-art facilities and information systems, and positive reputation in the market. If during this process you identify weaknesses in certain areas, begin to develop mechanisms to improve these areas.

Once your strengths have been identified, information should be compiled for use during contract negotiations to document these strengths. Exhibit 1.1 indicates the types of data to be collected, by category.

It is important to understand that payors with whom you negotiate have themselves collected information about you during their process of identifying potential network providers and preparing for negotiations. Payors must generally rely on publicly available information about providers, so you should review that data as well, to determine the accuracy and understand how the payor might perceive your strengths and weaknesses. When compiling your data, be sure to address any issues that may understate your strengths.

To substantiate your strategy, you should also gather information about competing providers, employers, and physicians in your market area. Exhibit 1.2 outlines the types of data to be collected about each group.

EXHIBIT 1.1. DATA ABOUT YOUR ORGANIZATION.

Type of Arrangement	Analyses to Perform:
Financial viability	Financial statements Financial indicators (strength of balance sheet) • Debt coverage ratio • Days cash on hand • Days in receivables • Asset turnover
Operations	Service mix Centers of excellence Payor mix by service Case mix intensity by service by payor Length of stay by service by payor Occupancy or capacity
Cost profile	Cost-to-charge ratios by major service Fixed and variable costs per procedure or case Capital costs Uncompensated care Teaching costs
Pricing structure	Charge Competitor charges
Other	Size Facilities Location Existing networks and affiliations Reputation with consumers (employers and employees) Reputation with other providers Information systems

Evaluate Potential Managed Care Partners

Finally, you also want to learn something about the managed care organizations in your market area to determine their relative strengths and whether their goals and activities are compatible with those of your organization. These questions can be used as a preliminary evaluation of managed care plans:

Reimbursement levels. Is the proposed reimbursement level generally acceptable? What is the method (discounted fee for service, per diem, per case, capitation), and how much risk is involved? Is the proposed amount negotiable?

EXHIBIT 1.2. DATA ABOUT YOUR MARKET.

Party	Have You Collected:
Competing providers	Market share Patient origin Range of services Payor affiliations Provider affiliations Medical staff composition • by specialty • by age • by practice arrangement (i.e., solo or group) Consumer preferences Technology: strengths and needs
Employer or customers	Local profile Size (number of employees) Industry (risk) Hospital utilization patterns Organized labor Current benefit offerings Perceptions and needs (market research findings) Price Service M.D. choice Hospital choice Employee residence Disposition to change
Physicians	Medical staff composition • Own and competitors' Attitudes toward managed care Formal organization and degree of integration Recruitment • Plans and history Physician support Objectives Composition of network • Specialty or location Credentialing to subscribers Risk-sharing arrangements

EXHIBIT 1.3. DETAILED PLAN ANALYSIS.

I. Control

   A. Sponsor
- Who organized this plan?
- Is it a subsidiary or new venture of a larger entity?

   B. Ownership
- Are the owners for-profit or not-for-profit?
- Who owns the plan?

   C. Board composition
- How many members are on the board?
- Does any particular group control it?
- Is a board seat available to your hospital or provider group?

   D. Profit sharing
- If the plan is profitable, will the hospital or its affiliated physicians benefit?

II. Marketing

   A. Target physicians
- Are particular groups of physicians being asked to participate?
- What are the criteria for selection of physicians?
- Is adequate geographic and specialty coverage provided?
- Which medical groups are associated with the plan?
- Which specialties are represented?

   B. Target patients
- What size employer groups are to be targeted?
- Will individually contracted, Medicare, or Medicaid patients be included?

   C. Target hospitals
- What are the plan's criteria for hospital selection? Does your hospital meet these criteria?
- Which are the participating hospitals in the plan's network?
- Are the other hospitals that have been approached, or are participating, cost-effective? (per day? per stay? per DRG?)
- Are specialty carveouts or globally priced products being offered?
- Do hospitals in the network pose a competitive threat to your facility?
- Could the plan use hospitals in the network to leverage your facility?
- Has the plan entered into any exclusive arrangement with other hospitals for specific services or geographic coverage?

   D. Marketing plan
- What are the plan's major group accounts?
- Does the plan have any guaranteed accounts? Where are they located? Are any of the accounts located in your hospital's service area?

(Continued)

EXHIBIT 1.3. Continued.

- What are the plan's types of employers (e.g., service, manufacturing, retail, etc.)?
- Is the marketing emphasis on large, medium, or small groups?
- How many members are enrolled in the plan?
- What are the plan's enrollment projections?
- What are the demographic characteristics of the expected enrollment?
- What is the plan's attrition or turnover rate?
- What has been the plan's actual membership growth rate to date? Is the plan's market share increasing?

E. Benefit package, services, copayments, deductibles
- What is the proposed benefit package? How does it compare to that of other plans in the area?
- If a PPO, is there sufficient financial incentive for the enrollees to use the preferred provider?

F. Education
- How is information to be communicated to enrollees?
- Are member materials clear and concise?

III. Reputation

- What is the plan's reputation?
- Do you expect affiliation with the plan to benefit or hurt the institution's reputation?
- Should your hospital become involved in the plan's advertising efforts?

IV. Financial

A. Capital contributions
- What capital contributions, if any, are required from participating providers?
- What control accompanies the contribution?
- Is the initial capital going to be adequate to finance development of the plan?

B. Physician reimbursement
- How are physicians compensated under this program?
- Are there incentives to encourage appropriate utilization patterns and discourage under- or overutilization?

C. Hospital payment
- What payment method is requested?
- Does the hospital have flexibility in the method used?
- Does the plan have a history of retroactively denying payment because of noncompliance with the utilization management process?

D. Hospital experience
- Is an incentive available to the hospital for favorable experience?
- What risk does the plan take for its actuarial assumptions?

- Is reinsurance or catastrophic stop-loss insurance a component of the risk arrangement?
- How is interest income handled on risk fund accounts?

E. Copayments
- Are copayments included?
- Is collection of copayments an administrative burden?

F. Coordination of benefits (COB)
- Who is responsible for collecting coordination-of-benefits revenue?
- Who has ownership of the revenue?
- Who is responsible for COB recovery costs?

G. Financial performance
- Does the plan process claims within contract provision time frames?
- If there have been payment delays, are they increasing or decreasing?
- Does the plan exhibit extreme conservatism in its claim disputes?
- Does the plan have problems maintaining accurate records on enrollee claims?
- Is the plan's utilization review poorly coordinated?
- Is the plan willing to consider a draft or periodic interim payment system?

H. Premium
- What premiums does the plan charge?
- How competitive is the premium with other plans in your area?
- Is the portion allocated to physician and hospital services reasonable?
- What utilization assumption is being made on hospital days per thousand enrollees?
- Is it perceived that the plan is attempting to "buy" membership in the first few years? If so, what may be the subsequent ramifications?

V. Medical

A. Utilization review
- Is an effective utilization review program included?
- How much review is the hospital responsible for performing?
- Are approvals required prior to delivery of services?

B. Quality assurance
- Can the plan provide appropriate data for peer review activities?
- How is patient satisfaction monitored?

C. Judgment and flexibility
- Does the plan limit involvement of surgical assistants, anesthetists, or nurse clinicians?
- Does the plan have the authority to retroactively deny claims?
- Under what circumstances could your hospital be dropped from the provider panel?

D. Malpractice risk implications
- Are you asked to indemnify other parties?

(Continued)

EXHIBIT 1.3. Continued.

- Is the professional judgment of your professional staff being limited without reduction of risk?
- Is the hospital contractually liable for physician acts?

E. Gatekeeper
- Is a "gatekeeper" part of the plan?
- When does this individual have to preauthorize services?

F. Specialist services
- Are specialty services limited to participating providers?
- Is a different reimbursement schedule used for specialty services?

G. Contract services (e.g., laboratory)
- Are laboratory or radiology services centralized?
- Will you be denied ancillary revenues?

VI. Management

A. Management team
- Who are the key management personnel?
- What education and experience do they have?
- Do they have a proven track record?
- How much management depth exists?
- Who will be the medical director?

B. Administrative costs
- What percentage of revenues is being set aside for administrative expense?
- What services are being provided for that fee?

C. Claims processing
- Does the plan have an effective claims processing system in place?
- How accurate is the data?
- Who processes claims: PPO, HMO, employer or Third Party Administrator (TPA), insurer?
- What is the claims turnaround time?

D. Management information system (MIS) capability
- Is the plan's MIS compatible with your internal system?
- Can the MIS generate data specific to your organization (e.g., utilization, cost, quality, physician profiling, and contract management capabilities)?

VII. Licensure

- Is the plan licensed by an appropriate state regulatory body?
- Is the HMO federally qualified?
- What are the implications of contracting with either a qualified or a nonqualified plan (e.g., state reserve requirements, experience versus adjusted community rating)?

VIII. Hospital utilization

- Can the plan provide utilization statistics (i.e., age, sex, acuity level, volume) and experience summaries regarding the plan's membership?
- What do you see in comparing the plan's current utilization rate (admissions per thousand members per month) with rates projected under the contract terms?
- Have the plan's actuarial assumptions been obtained and reviewed for reasonableness as they relate to the proposed contract?
- If your hospital already has most of the plan's business (employer groups, PPOs), does your hospital gain incremental volume by contracting at a new discount rate, or does your hospital cannibalize an existing payor segment?
- Is the plan's utilization management program physician-driven or member-driven?
- What are the plan's intentions to use the hospital's ancillary services (home health, urgent care, etc.)?

IX. Medicare risk

- Has the plan entered, or will it enter, into a Medicare risk contract with the U.S. Health Care Financing Administration (HCFA)?
- If so, does the plan believe it will profit from this contract?
- What impact does the Medicare risk contract have on the proposed relationship between the plan and hospital? (E.g., will utilization increase? Are additional provisions required? Are there any other billing or collection requirements?)

X. Medicaid risk

- Has the plan entered, or will it enter, into a Medicaid risk contract with the state/HCFA?
- If so, does the plan believe it will profit from this contract?
- What impact does the Medicaid risk contract have on the proposed relationship between the plan and hospital? (E.g., will utilization increase? Are additional provisions required? Are there any other billing or collection requirements?)

Source: Reprinted, by permission, from *Healthcare Financial Management*, May 1986, p. 41. Copyright ©1986 by the HEALTHCARE FINANCIAL MANAGEMENT ASSOCIATION

Marketability. Does the managed care plan have an existing track record in your area? Are you interested in this market segment? Does the plan have advance commitments from accounts? If so, for how many enrollees?

Effect on existing business. Are you likely to lose business if you do not contract with this plan? What is the plan's historical volume with your organization? Are your patients likely to change coverage if you do not become a participating provider? Will your medical staff participate in the plan even if the hospital chooses not to?

Enrollment guarantees. Are enrollment guarantees offered? If so, how many patients are guaranteed?

Commitment. What level of commitment is required? Is termination flexible for you? For the other party?

Other providers. Have other providers also been approached by the managed care plan? If so, are you comfortable with these "partners"?

If your preliminary analysis results in favorable assessment, you may want to perform more detailed analysis before making a final decision about entering into a contractual arrangement with the managed care plan. Exhibit 1.3 presents the components of an appropriate detailed plan analysis.

Exhibit 1.4 identifies the types of information you should gather about local managed care payors.

EXHIBIT 1.4. INFORMATION ABOUT MANAGED CARE ORGANIZATIONS.

Data Category	Data to Be Collected
Operations	Market share Patient origin Range of services List of provider affiliations Physician network structure • by specialty • do they target certain types of M.D.s? • Solo or group
Financial viability	Financial statements • strength of balance sheet • net worth
Cost structure	Medical loss ratio Administrative cost ratio • Marketing cost ratio
Pricing structure	Premium structure • compared to other managed care payors in market • historical growth relative to market
Employer profile	List of accounts in local market and penetration in each Target prospects Marketing plan for region • strategy • market mix and budget • time frames and targets Experience in other markets Distinct competitive advantages Local market research Consumer satisfaction

	• disenrollment rates
	• relative satisfaction
	Member demographics (age-and-sex mix, top diagnoses, hospital utilization by service)
Physicians	Composition of network
	Information to subscribers
	Risk-sharing arrangements with hospital and plan
	Practice supports available

Assign Negotiating Team

Finally, your plan should identify a team of individuals responsible for reviewing or assisting in negotiating the contract. This team should include experienced legal and financial professionals.

If your organization does not have the relevant expertise to handle contract negotiations, consider involving appropriate outside professional resources, such as attorneys, accountants, consultants, and actuaries. Responsibility for negotiating and coordinating external and internal managed care activities should be delegated to a single individual. This same individual should be given sufficient authority to respond quickly to contracting opportunities and service problems.

In developing your managed care contracting strategy, it is important to involve individuals from operational areas (admitting, business office, accounting, nursing, utilization review) that are affected by the contract. These individuals can identify specific operational limitations or other contractual concerns that should be reflected in the negotiating position. Once contract terms have been proposed, these same individuals should review and approve those terms that affect their areas of responsibility.

CHAPTER TWO

DEVELOPING A CONTRACTING STRATEGY

Developing a contracting strategy involves two phases. In the first phase, a provider must assess its historic mission and strategic goals and translate them into a tactical plan that highlights its organizational strengths. The second phase would have the provider organization comparing its strategy to the marketplace needs of a specific managed care organization from the viewpoint of its own cachet in the market, payor mix, and market share. Because a provider's contracting strategy may involve developing and issuing a request for proposal, this chapter also offers guidance on writing an RFP.

The risk contracting process usually begins when a managed care organization presents a contract to a provider to sign. Since the managed care organization is familiar with the contract and probably has used it before, it is likely to have a definite advantage. However, you can balance the situation by developing, in advance, a contracting strategy to guide you through the negotiation process.

Contracting strategy is a function of your organizational objectives and negotiating strength relative to those of the managed care organization. The ultimate goal of a contract negotiation is to achieve a win-win situation in which both provider and payor walk away with contract terms that satisfy each one's business objectives. To achieve this end, you must go into the negotiation with a keen understanding of not only your own goals and objectives, strengths, and weaknesses but also those of your "opponent." (Use of the term *opponent* is perhaps inappropriate since, subsequent to a successful negotiation, the other party is ideally seen as more like a "partner.")

Developing a contracting strategy simply involves tailoring your action plan into a strategy that matches your goals, objectives, and unique strengths to the needs of a specific managed care organization.

Competitive Factors

There are four important factors that apply to evaluating the synergy between a prospective provider participant and a managed care organization.

Market Share

Much of the strength of either party is based on respective market share. A managed care plan that is solidly established in the area and holds a large membership may have leverage over a provider because of its control over demand for health care services. A plan that is new or has few subscribers possesses comparatively little negotiating clout. Likewise, a provider that has significant market dominance may be in a stronger negotiating position for managed care business than its competitors in the region.

Nature of the Targeted Market

Health plans often seek to develop particular markets, as defined by type of patient, geographic location, or service niche. For example, many managed care plans are interested in developing Medicare risk products and may therefore be more willing to negotiate favorable terms with a hospital that serves a large Medicare population. Or perhaps a plan needs to provide obstetric services in a particular geographic region. Again, a hospital may be able to win concessions from a plan if it can meet a particular need.

Reputation

By nature, organizations seek to affiliate with others that are well respected in the market. From the work performed in developing a plan for managed care contracting, you should already know what your reputation is in the market, as well as that of the plan.

Clearly, a provider that has a reputation for quality patient care and strong financial results and has accessible location(s) is in a stronger negotiating position than providers with weaker reputations. Likewise, payors known for ensuring quality care to their membership and for treating providers fairly are most attractive to providers seeking contractual relationships with managed care organizations.

Leverage

As a rule, the participant with the strongest market share and reputation has the greatest leverage at the negotiating table. Payors often leverage their negotiation as well by limiting the number of providers they bring into their network. This approach could work to the payor's disadvantage, however, to the extent that it does not have the appropriate provider network to meet the demand of their membership. A provider can exert leverage in these situations if it is able to attract the support of major accounts in the payor market.

Requests for Proposal

The contracting process usually begins when a managed care organization presents a proposed contract or issues an RFP to the provider.

Managed care organizations most frequently use RFPs when selectivity within the network delivery system is introduced. However, in those markets where the managed care organizations contract with the vast majority of physicians and hospitals, RFPs are seldom used. The MCOs annually engage in contract renewals based upon their ongoing profile of each provider. In some cases, however, if the provider is in a position of relative strength in the marketplace, RFPs may be issued from the provider to the managed care plan.

An RFP and responses typically follow a structure that includes specific types of information. The information given to the potential respondents to the RFP generally highlights these topics:

- Brief description of organization
- Description of arrangements or services sought
- Clearly and concisely stated information requirements
- Deadline for submission
- Criteria upon which the selection is to be made
- Name and address of individual to whom response should be directed
- Contact person
- Timing of the final selection
- Means of notification

Brief Description of Organization

This section generally includes a basic profile. Hospitals, for example, include the number of inpatient beds and special services, such as a trauma center, burn center, pediatric emergency room, perinatal center, intensive care units, and subspecialty clinics. Patient mix, accreditation status (for example, certification by the Joint Commission on the Accreditation of Healthcare Organizations, or JCAHO), and the service area are usually included, in addition to the number of employees and number of physicians. Further information on financial condition and any ongoing merger discussions is also generally disclosed.

Physician practice groups describe their professional services. For example, multispecialty group practices delineate the specialty care provided (OB/GYN, cardiology, internal medicine, gastroenterology, etc.). Participation with a JCAHO-accredited hospital, board certification, or board eligibility of physicians in specialty areas along with the number of physicians, number of employees, service area, and approximate number of patient office visits per year would also be included in a brief description.

In an RFP from a managed care organization, brief description of the organization includes the service area and number of members, among other basic information (product offerings, NCQA—National Committee on Quality Assurance—status, financial standing, business and strategic plans, network providers, discount arrangements, payment methodologies, medical management programs, quality initiatives, and so on).

Description of Arrangements or Services Sought

Brief description of the purpose of the RFP includes the arrangement or services sought. For example, an organization may be seeking a risk-sharing contract for professional clinical services. The potential for risk sharing includes hospital risk pools, an incentive program relative to management of a teaching program, and achievement of clinical outcome measurements.

Clearly and Concisely Stated Information Requirements

An RFP generally asks responders to describe their approach, for example, to managed care risk contracting and capitation arrangements and to provide details on market-specific knowledge. Pertinent questions on how an organization administers such functions as credentialing, outcomes data capture and compliance, disease management, case management, and customer service and appeals may also be included. Sample contracts with similarly situated organizations, inpatient and outpatient service categories and proposed rates and billing requirements, and brief biographies of key individuals within an organization are also typically requested.

Deadline for Submission

Most RFPs are complex documents. Even so, the time for response to an RFP can vary from a few days to a few weeks.

Criteria upon Which the Selection Is Made

The RFP should describe how the information you have requested is evaluated and weighed in making the final decision. For example, what is more important: discounts, quality, or broadness of the network? There may be some discussion of a "first cut" that produces a list of "finalists." A bidders' conference may be held to provide opportunity for discussion surrounding the RFP. In some cases, responders are asked to make an in-person presentation.

Name and Address of Individual to Whom Response Should Be Directed

The name and address, phone number, and e-mail address of the individual to whom responses to the RFP need to be directed should be clearly stated. If a committee is evaluating the RFP, it is convenient to provide multiple copies of the RFP reply for all committee members.

Contact Person

Many organizations designate a contact person to handle questions regarding the RFP, including clarification of the information requirements, deadline extensions, and other issues.

Timing of the Final Selection

Review of responses to RFP submissions typically requires two to four weeks. However, the timing may be accelerated depending upon an organization's own urgency to reach a decision. It is likely that the selection process will involve a certain amount of negotiation by both parties.

Means of Notification

Notification to applicants of the final decision regarding an RFP is generally made in writing. Execution of an agreement that contains specific performance expectations, guarantees, and penalties concludes the contracting process.

CHAPTER THREE

EVALUATING A PROPOSAL

Evaluating a proposal from a managed care organization should focus on its most critical components: the payment arrangement and the degree of risk for the provider. Understanding and evaluating the degree of risk is essential to tailoring a sound risk contract.

Perhaps the most critical component of a managed care contract is the payment arrangement. Payment arrangements in contracts between providers and payors can take a variety of forms. Unless the contract is based on full cost, you are required to accept some degree of financial risk. The nature and degree of that risk varies depending on the unit of service and the basis for payment.

Overview of Payment Arrangements

Figure 3.1 illustrates how risk is shifted from insurer to provider according to differing payment arrangements. The following describes types of payment arrangements and the risks associated with each.

Fee-for-Service (Price Risk)

Fee-for-service payment arrangements may be based on an agreed-upon discount from charges, or on a fee schedule for services rendered. Providers that accept

FIGURE 3.1. RISK CONTINUUM.

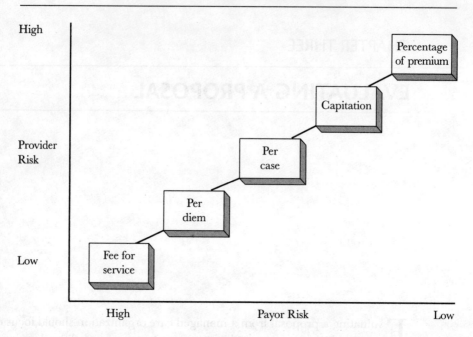

fee-for-service payment arrangements risk the possibility that payment rates do not cover variable costs and make an inadequate contribution to overhead. This is known as *price risk*.

Fee schedules may be based on "reasonable and customary" charges in a provider's service area. Sometimes a payor may use a relative value scale arrangement, which ties payment for services to the relative weight of those services. A common example is the Medicare Resource-Based Relative Value Scale (RBRVS) fee schedule used to reimburse physicians. The relative weight is based on the resources consumed, as determined by such factors as personnel time, level of skill, and sophistication of equipment required to render the services.

Managed care plans tend to use fee-for-service arrangements if the plan does not represent a significant amount of business to the provider. As the plan achieves greater market penetration and providers rely more heavily on that payor for a significant percentage of revenue, other payment arrangements are often applied to shift greater risk to the provider.

Per Diem (Intensity Risk)

A managed care contract may require you to aggregate individual services into average daily rates and accept a per diem rate as payment in full. In this situation, the hospital assumes an *intensity risk* because it must correctly estimate its average costs and the volume and mix of services it provides each day. Analyses show that inpatients receive the most intense treatment during their first few days of hospitalization. A contracted per diem rate that represents a calculated average daily rate may be below actual cost in the first days of hospitalization, and higher than cost in the last days of care. If the hospital's average length of stay decreases to below that assumed in the negotiated rate, total payment for the case may not be sufficient to cover total cost. Patients enrolled in the managed care plan may require a greater volume of ancillary services each day, and the cost to the hospital of providing those services may be higher than anticipated. Because these contracts do not allow for retrospective adjustments if actual intensity is greater than expected, the hospital may lose money.

Health plans often use per diem arrangements in the early phases of managed care to take advantage of the savings to be realized as the length of stay is reduced.

Per Case (Price, Intensity, and Severity Risk)

Hospitals may also contract on a per case basis. This is similar to the Medicare DRG system, although patient categories can be defined differently. In addition to price risk and intensity risk, hospitals that contract on a per case basis accept *severity risk*. Because hospitals are paid an average flat price per discharge category, the risk is that the total cost of services actually required by an individual patient could potentially exceed the revenue earmarked for that patient. Since the payment remains constant regardless of length of stay or total cost of care, under per case payment the risk to a hospital is likely to be greater than under per diem payment arrangements. However, to the extent that length of stay can be reduced, the opportunity for gain can also be greater.

Global pricing is a form of per case pricing that incorporates not only payment to the hospital for its services but also payment to the physician for professional services.

Capitation (Price, Intensity, Severity, and Frequency Risk)

Under capitation, a provider is paid a flat amount each month for each health plan enrollee that is a member of the provider's assigned population. In return for this capitation payment, the provider assumes the obligation to provide all medical services required by enrollees as defined by the specified covered-benefits list.

For example, a hospital might contract with an HMO to provide all necessary inpatient acute and critical care, nursing home and rehabilitative care, home health care, and all emergency room care for a specified population for $35 per member per month. Under this arrangement, in addition to all other risks defined above, the hospital assumes a *frequency risk*. In other words, the hospital is at risk for all overall use rates of the specific population assigned to the hospital.

Percentage of Premium (Price, Intensity, Severity, Frequency, and Actuarial or Marketing Risk)

Percentage of premium and capitation arrangements are very similar in that both are based on prepayment of a periodic amount in exchange for the obligation to provide defined health care services to a specified population. Percentage of premium contracts, however, expose the provider to an additional element of risk. Under percentage of premium contracts, the payor agrees to give a predetermined percentage of its monthly premiums to the provider to cover the total cost of medical services for a defined population. Since payment to the provider depends on both the number of subscribers and the premium charged to subscribers, in addition to other risks the provider is also exposed to an *actuarial or marketing risk*.

For example, premiums charged by a managed care plan may prove to be too low if the enrollee's actual family size is larger than anticipated. A larger family is likely to result in higher than budgeted medical service costs per family contract. Similarly, a plan might be forced to reduce premiums in response to market competition. In either case, provider revenue is directly affected and can be below actual cost. Unlike capitation contracts, percentage of premium arrangements force providers to bear some of the risk for the managed care plan's actuarial assumptions and marketing strategy. In today's highly competitive and ever-changing environment, this type of contract is likely to be the riskiest for providers.

Figure 3.2 outlines the risks and critical variables associated with the different types of payment arrangements.

Figure 3.3 distinguishes the contracting risk factors by type of payment arrangement for the provider versus the managed care payor.

Evaluating the Financial Arrangement

The first step in quantifying the financial impact of the contract is to identify how services are defined, who is responsible for providing the services, and how compensation is determined. Analyzing a capitation arrangement is much more complex than analyzing a discounted fee-for-service arrangement. Particularly with capitated contracts, care should be exercised to ensure that responsibilities for nonhospital services are well understood. In some situations, a hospital may be responsible for any medical services required to be rendered to plan members, such as for long-term care, chemical dependency, and home health care.

FIGURE 3.2. VARIABLES AFFECTING RISK.

Level of Risk	Contract Type	Nature of Risk	Critical Variables
Low	Discounted charge	Price	Contribution margin (Price − variable cost) × volume
	Per diem	Price	Contribution margin
		Intensity	Volume of ancillary services per patient
			Mix of days by unit
	Per case (global pricing)	Price	Contribution margin
		Intensity	Volume of ancillary services per patient
			Mix of days by unit
		Severity	Length of stay
	Capitation	Price	Contribution margin
		Intensity	Volume of ancillary services per patient
			Mix of days by unit
		Severity	Length of stay
		Frequency	Admission rate
			Out-of-hospital claims costs
	Percentage of premium	Price	Contribution margin
		Intensity	Volume of ancillary services per patient
			Mix of days by unit
		Severity	Length of stay
		Frequency	Admission rate
			Out-of-hospital claims costs
		Actuarial	Average contract size
High		Marketing	HMO marketing strategy

FIGURE 3.3. CONTRACT RISK FACTORS
BY TYPE OF PAYMENT ARRANGEMENT.

Payment Arrangement	Utilization	Unit Cost	Age and Sex of Membership	Benefit Design
Fee-for-service	P	P	P	P
Per diem	P	H	P if days ↑ H if intensity ↑	P
Per case	P	H	H if days ↑ or if intensity ↑	P
Capitation • PMPM	H	H	H	P
• by age and sex	H	H	P	P
• by contract type	H	H	H	H

H = hospital is at risk
P = managed care plan is at risk

A hospital without adequate cost data may find it very difficult to determine the costs of these services.

Once the general nature of the arrangement is understood, you should try to estimate the volume you will receive from the contract and identify costs associated with providing the agreed-upon care. The accuracy of the estimates depends largely on the availability and quality of the underlying data. Regardless of the proposed payment arrangement, the provider should identify its cost of providing care under a contract. Accurate cost information should be collected and made available to key management decision makers. Let us examine the cost information needed to evaluate a proposed contract or assess the profitability of an existing contract.

Cost Per Procedure

Many health care providers lack a sophisticated cost accounting system, which is necessary to determine procedure-level costs with a fine degree of accuracy. As an alternative, this information may be determined using a departmentwide ratio of cost to charges, a relative value scale, or a standard cost approach. Costs should be broken into fixed and variable components.

Cost or Revenue Per Case

Actual resources consumed in treating patients should be determined using previously identified procedure-cost information. Revenue information for noncapitated patients should also be gathered. This type of information is often collected through a hospital's revenue, case mix reporting, or cost accounting systems.

Product, Product Line, and Market Information

Patient-level data should be aggregated into product groups such as DRGs, disease stage categories, or APGs (ambulatory procedure groups), which are then aggregated into product line (such as women's and children's health, oncology, plastic surgery, ENT services) and markets (as by payor, employer, or age groups).

The amount of detail desired may depend on the nature of the payment arrangement. For example, market level information by age or sex is important in evaluating capitation contracts. However, evaluations of discounted charge contracts may require only procedure cost information.

Next, you should determine the effect of the contract on profitability. Generally, a contribution margin approach is useful. Contribution margin is defined as:

$$(\text{PRICE} - \text{VARIABLE COST}) \times \text{VOLUME}$$

An analysis that does not consider all three of these variables is incomplete and may lead to an incorrect decision. It is important to understand the distinction between full cost and variable cost. Even though the offered price is less than the full cost of the service (variable cost plus allocated fixed cost), if the contribution margin is positive (price exceeds the variable cost) it is profitable for the provider to render the service.

Exhibit 3.1 summarizes the key components and information appropriate for analysis of each type of financial arrangement.

A final factor to consider, particularly in capitation contracting, is the impact the contract has on cash flow. Generally, you should be able to negotiate rapid payment terms, and interest penalties for slow payment. Capitation goes a step further and reverses the traditional financial cycle by requiring payment in advance of the time medical services are rendered. Also, under most managed care capitation arrangements, patient copays and deductibles are reduced or eliminated, which greatly reduces bad debt.

EXHIBIT 3.1. METHODOLOGIES TO EVALUATE PAYMENT.

Type of Arrangement	Analyses to Perform
Discounted charges	• Determine cost for services covered by proposed rate. May need to separate inpatient and outpatient costs, and costs by type of service. • If costs determined above represent an average for all patients treated, adjust for estimated acuity of type of patient covered by managed care plan, i.e., Medicare patients require higher intensity of treatment and longer length of stay on average than commercial indemnity patients. A patient enrolled in a PPO is more likely to use more services than a patient in a tightly managed HMO. • Allocate costs between fixed and variable. • Estimate volume you expect from this payor. • Calculate contribution margin: (Price – Variable cost) × Volume. As long as contribution margin is positive, the rate is profitable. • Compare rate to rates paid by other payors to determine whether it is competitive in your market.
Per diem	• Estimate average cost per day by type of service adjusted for estimated acuity of patient type. • Allocate costs between fixed and variable. • Estimate volume in terms of days (admissions × ALOS) by type of service. • Calculate the weighted average cost per day for all services. • Calculate contribution margin. *Additional analyses:* • Calculate average cost per case for this type of patient. Divide by estimated ALOS and compare result to proposed per diem rate for reasonableness. • Estimate how much LOS may be reduced through utilization management by the payor. Ensure that per diem rate is adequate to cover cost even if LOS is reduced. • Restate rate as a percentage of charges, and compare to rates paid by other payors. • Consider negotiating a "tiered rate" that is higher for the first days of an inpatient stay to recognize the greater intensity of treatment typically delivered in the first few days of hospitalization.
Per case	• Determine average cost per case adjusted for estimated acuity of patient type. (Note: some payors, i.e., Medicare, base payment on a case mix neutral rate adjusted on a per case basis for the acuity of the particular patient as determined by the assigned

diagnoses and procedure codes. This helps to reduce the possibility of a per case payment being significantly above or below cost.)
- Allocate costs between fixed and variable.
- Estimate volume expected from this payor in terms of number of discharges.
- Calculate the weighted average cost per case for all services.
- Calculate contribution margin.

Additional analyses:

- Determine assumed LOS that underlies the rate. Be certain the case can be managed to that LOS.
- Consider negotiating different rates by type of service (e.g., medical or surgical, ICU or CCU, obstetrics) to recognize differences in cost.
- If volume from this payor is expected to be low, consider negotiating a higher rate for the first X number of cases, with a discounted rate for all cases past the designated volume threshold.

Capitation
- Identify specific services covered by capitation rate. This is defined by the managed care payor's benefit plan for the particular insurance product offered.
- Determine which covered services can be provided by participating providers in your organization versus those that you do not perform and thus must be referred.
- Obtain historical utilization data by type of service. This is expressed as units of service/1,000 members and should be available from the plan as generated by their claims processing system. For inpatient utilization, determine ALOS by service.
- Estimate how utilization may change under a more tightly managed system. An actuary can help with these estimates.
- Estimate cost by type of service.
- Calculate cost per unit of service by dividing cost by utilization/1,000 members.
- Obtain payor's assumed price per unit of service that is built into the capitation rate.
- Compare payor's price per unit of service to actual cost per unit.
- Compare historical reimbursement rates (per day, per case) expressed on a per unit of service basis to the assumed prices/unit that underlie the capitation rate.
- Define noncovered and excluded services to determine those services for which you are not responsible and may bill fee-for-service or refer patients to other providers for treatment.

Special Issues Related to Capitation

Capitation is unlike any other form of payment arrangement in that it totally reverses the financial incentives to physicians and hospitals. Table 3.1 presents the varying financial incentives that underlie each of the payment arrangements. Note that only under capitation are hospital and physician incentives fully aligned. Under other forms of payment arrangements, the incentives for the hospital may be at odds with the physician's. Table 3.2 illustrates how incentives are altered when payment arrangements migrate from fee-for-service to riskier arrangements such as per diem or per case payment and, finally, capitation.

Payors may prefer capitation arrangements because they motivate providers to deliver cost-effective medical care and make the payor's costs more predictable. By paying the provider a fixed amount per member per month, most of the risk

TABLE 3.1. IMPACT OF USE RATES ON PAYMENT ARRANGEMENTS.

Hospital Incentives

Payment Arrangement	Admissions	Patient Days	Ancillary Services
Reasonable and customary fee for service, charges	+	+	+
Discounted fee for services	++	++	++
Per diem	+	++	–
Per case (DRG)	++	–	–
Capitation	–	–	–

Physician Incentives

Payment Arrangement	Physician Services	Hospital Admissions	Hospital Patient Days
Reasonable and customary fee for service	+	+	+
Discounted fee for service	++	++	++
Fee for service with withholds and risk pools	++ to neutral	+	Neutral
Per case (DRG)	–	++	–
Capitation with risk pool	–	–	–

+ (and ++) = Increased use rate, positive financial impact
– = Decreased use rate, negative financial impact

of unanticipated utilization and higher costs are borne by the provider. The payor is able to predetermine its costs and thereby project profit with more certainty.

The provider's willingness to accept the greater risks associated with capitation depends on its position and experience in the market. A provider with declining utilization in a competitive market may be willing to enter a capitation contract as a means of maintaining market share. On the other hand, a dominant community provider may be more resistant to accepting the risks associated with capitation.

Capitation arrangements are the most difficult to evaluate because of the complexity of the variables involved in developing the rate. You might consider employing the services of an actuary who can build assumptions about the future to estimate the results of accepting a given capitation rate. Specifically, an actuary seeks to estimate:

- Expected cost per member
- Variation in cost based on plan benefit
- Age and sex characteristics of member population
- Expected cost by type of provider

Actuarial studies may also be used to develop price and utilization targets and to determine how to allocate the capitation rate among providers. A typical actuarial model reflects assumptions about membership demographics, plan design, utilization of network services and out-of-network services, cost per unit of service

TABLE 3.2. TRANSFORMATION OF FINANCIAL INCENTIVES.

	Yesterday	Today	Tomorrow
Common payment arrangements	Cost base Fee for service	Per diem Per case Fee for service Capitation	Capitation

Hospital incentives	High occupancy
	High charges
	High utilization
			Increase
			  covered lives
			Reduce
			  admissions, days,
			  ancillaries
			Control cost

Physician incentives	Medical
	  intervention
	Generate volume
			Medical
			  management
			Increase covered
			  lives
			Reduce volume
			Control cost

(based on expected physician and facility fees), levels of reinsurance, coordination of benefits, and plan administrative expenses and profit targets. Table 3.3 presents a sample capitation budget that includes these factors.

Methods of Limiting Risk

When a contract entails significant financial risks, it may be advantageous to consider ways to limit those risks. There are several techniques in common use with capitation contracts. As with all other components of the financial arrangement, these methods of limiting risk should be described fully in the contract.

Reinsurance, Stop-Loss

These techniques are used to guard against the risk that unforeseen and unpredictable events pose for demand and cost of health care services. Variables such as the appearance of new diseases or epidemics, new technology breakthroughs, or changes in governmental regulations could result in major problems for a provider under a capitation contract.

A common way to limit the risk of unforeseen or unusual demand under a risk contract is with reinsurance coverage. Reinsurance (or stop-loss coverage) is like any other type of insurance policy in which a defined benefit level is provided for a predetermined premium. Under capitation contracts, the payor frequently provides the reinsurance, sets the premium (and subtracts it from the monthly capitation payment to the provider), and determines the level of coverage. In some cases, providers can either purchase their own coverage on the open market or negotiate the terms of the coverage provided through the payor.

Stop-loss insurance may be written on an individual claim basis whereby any claim over a specified amount can be submitted to the carrier for payment. A *claim* is usually defined as all expenses incurred for covered benefits resulting from a single accident or episode of illness. This may be a single bill for an inpatient hospitalization, or it may be the sum of separate bills for ambulance, emergency room, hospital inpatient, rehabilitation, home health care, and so forth. (Stop-loss insurance is frequently written on the basis of the cost of total annual claims per individual. In this situation, the policy pays for all or a significant portion of covered expenses for an enrollee during the year in excess of a specified amount.)

Aggregate stop-loss insurance may also be purchased. Aggregate policies apply to all claims that are incurred by the provider during the contract term, not just to specific claims. For example, an aggregate policy might be obtained to cover claims expense in excess of $10 million.

TABLE 3.3. CAPITATION COMPONENT MODEL.

Service Category	Frequency (Units/1,000)	Average Cost per Unit	PMPM, $
Inpatient			
Obstetrics (including nursery)	74	$965	$5.95
Medical/surgical (including ICU and pediatric)	253	1,200	25.30
Nursing home care	10	225	0.19
Total inpatient			31.44
Physician, hospital outpatient, and other			
Office visit/M.D.	3,936	$48	$15.74
Psych outpatient visit/M.D.	620	56	2.89
Inpatient visit/M.D.	296	87	2.15
Psych inpatient visit/M.D.	5	104	.04
Home visit/M.D.	1	120	.01
Anesthesiologist/M.D.			4.00
Obstetrics/M.D.	59	855	4.20
Inpatient surgery/M.D.	63	647	3.40
Outpatient surgery/M.D.	398	159	5.27
Dental services	47	138	.54
Eye care	130	60	.65
Injections and immunizations	373	35	1.09
Therapies	476	49	1.94
Diagnostics	1,167	43	4.18
Lab	5,000	12	5.00
Radiology	1,400	100	11.67
Misc. physician services	330	37	1.02
Other outpatient department services	197	170	2.79
Emergency room	275	188	4.31
DME/supplies	38	168	.53
Day surgery	59	1,159	5.70
Home health care	141	116	1.36
Dialysis	11	273	.25
Total physician, hospital outpatient, and other			78.73

Definitions:
1. Frequency in units per thousand members = (total service units in the category) divided by (total members divided by 1,000)
2. Average cost per unit = total service category costs divided by total service category units
3. PMPM = (frequency in units per thousand members) multiplied by (average cost per unit divided by total member months)

You must decide in your negotiations with a payor, or in seeking reinsurance, what level of risk to retain. The greater the risk retained, the lower the cost of your reinsurance premium. After one or two years of actual claims experience, and with a properly designed decision support system, you should be able to determine the optimal risk-benefit tradeoff to maximize the net amount recovered through claims to the reinsurance carrier.

Withholds

Often, a payor may withhold a portion of the payments that are due the provider as a form of reserve against the possibility of budget excesses. If at the end of the contract period the provider has met budget, the withhold is returned. If the budget has been exceeded, the payor retains that portion of the withhold needed to cover the provider's budget deficit.

Carveouts

Providers may treat certain specialty types of cases that by their nature have high and unpredictable costs. Examples include HIV, neonatal, open heart surgery, or organ transplants. In some cases, the payor may agree to "carve out" these cases from the base capitation rate and pay for them under a separate arrangement (such as a discounted fee schedule or fixed case with outlier payments).

Risk Sharing

Another common way to limit risk is through establishing risk pools. Risk pools are arrangements by which physicians, payors, or both agree to share a portion of potential losses (or gains) that a provider might experience. Final payment is usually based on attaining an agreed-upon level of utilization. If actual utilization and costs are lower than expected, then the payor, the physician, and the hospital share in the savings. On the other hand, if utilization is higher than expected, all parties bear the extra cost.

Risk sharing arrangements range from fairly simple to extremely complex and may be used in combination with any compensation arrangement. The arrangements may spread the risk of excess cost, excess utilization, or both. The risk may or may not be shared equally among all parties. There may be limits on the maximum risk one of the participants assumes. There can also be multiple risk pools based on different incentives.

Providers must also determine how to allocate their share of the surplus or deficit among the participants in the risk pool. Generally, the participants include the hospital and primary care physicians (PCPs) and, in some cases, specialty care physicians.

Surplus or deficit may be shared in any fashion that supports the goals of the provider organization, and the basis for allocation may be multifaceted—that is, apportionment may be based partly on financial performance, partly on quality of care measures, and partly on patient satisfaction.

Generally, the payor wants to create risk pools not only to reduce its financial risk but also to create incentives for providers to control utilization. The hospital may be willing to participate in a risk pool to reduce its risk of loss from higher-than-expected costs and utilization. The physician might view participation as an opportunity to share in the financial rewards of an efficient health care program. Both the payor and the hospital want the primary care physician involved, since he or she can control access to medical services by acting as a gatekeeper to the health care system and is in the best position to control utilization. By tying the physician's payment to the cost of services rendered, the risk pool provides a strong financial incentive to the physician to control utilization and cost.

To illustrate the various principles of capitation contracting and risk sharing, Figures 3.4, 3.5, and 3.6 present three simple models of how a capitation payment may be allocated among hospital, primary care physicians, and specialty care physicians. It should be noted that these models are simply examples. Risk sharing arrangements may be designed to meet the specific objectives of the parties to the contract negotiation.

Table 3.4 presents a summary of current industry trends in physician compensation and surplus-deficit allocation methodologies. Table 3.5 presents a list of possible factors upon which to base the allocation of dollars.

As a final step in evaluating a capitation contract, you must ascertain your organization's ability to manage the unique risk inherent in this type of payment arrangement. Perform an internal assessment that addresses:

Strength of your utilization management. Under capitation, you must be able to move patients efficiently from the hospital to the most appropriate, cost-effective site of service. As part of this assessment, determine your facility's average length of stay by service line to identify areas of opportunity to reduce the duration of an inpatient stay.

Strength of relationships between hospital and physicians. Physicians are the ultimate decision makers when it comes to patient care. To achieve the efficiency of operations required for success under capitation, physicians must understand the incentives and dynamics of capitation arrangements, and all parties to the arrangement must work together.

FIGURE 3.4. RISK-SHARING MODEL:
FULL RISK-SHARING CAPITATION.

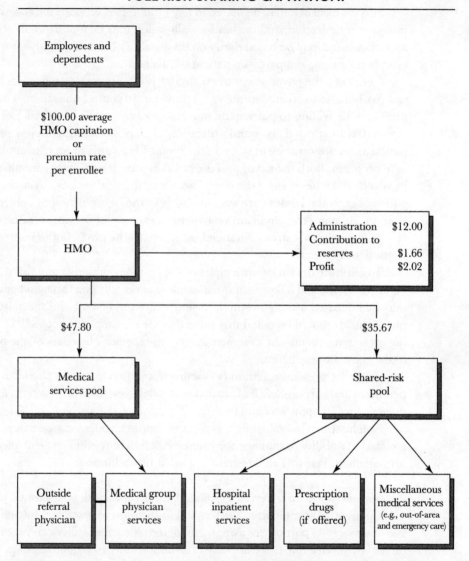

Employees and dependents

$100.00 average HMO capitation or premium rate per enrollee

HMO

Administration	$12.00
Contribution to reserves	$1.66
Profit	$2.02

$47.80

$35.67

Medical services pool

Shared-risk pool

Outside referral physician

Medical group physician services

Hospital inpatient services

Prescription drugs (if offered)

Miscellaneous medical services (e.g., out-of-area and emergency care)

Physician group risk: medical group is at full risk for physician services covered by the capitation payment, accepting total risk for referrals.

Risk sharing: physicians are to be paid by the HMO up to 15% of any surplus over the amounts disbursed from the shared-risk pool in each year, or pay to the HMO up to 15% of any deficits over the amount allocated to the shared-risk pool at the end of the year.

FIGURE 3.5. RISK-SHARING MODEL: PERCENTAGE OF PREMIUM CAPITATION.

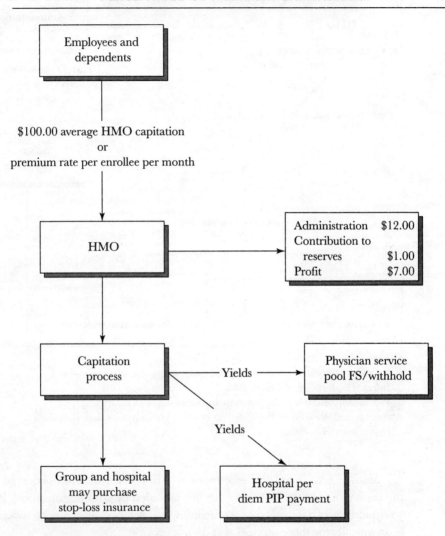

- If utilization target met, M.D.s share excess (55% PCPs, 45% specialists)
- If utilization target is exceeded, withholds are lost
- If hospital utilization exceeds target, PIP payment is lowered and physician withholds are forfeited
- If hospital utilization is less than target, PIP payment is higher and 50% of excess goes to physicians (55% to specialists, 45% PCPs)

FIGURE 3.6. RISK-SHARING MODEL: CARVE-OUT CAPITATION.

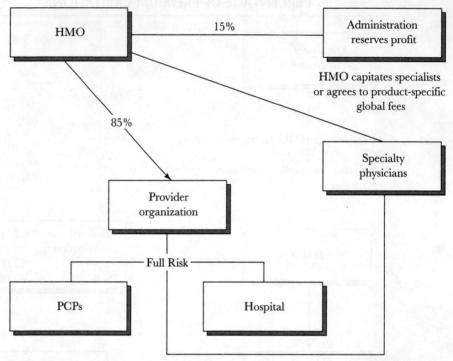

Features:
1. Based on capitation process, all providers are capitated, as is the hospital.
2. Internal budgets control funds flow.
3. Provider organization may purchase inpatient stop-loss insurance.
4. Any capitation excess or loss based on budgeted utilization is shared by the physicians and hospital.

Status of relationships with other providers. List all of the services covered under the capitation arrangement that are not provided by your organization. Review your patterns of referral to other facilities, and assess your ability to subcontract economically for those services you do not provide.

As depicted in Figure 3.4, suppose an HMO requires from employer groups, on behalf of their enrolled employees and dependents, an average first-year capitation or premium of $100 per enrollee per month to cover all operating costs. (It should be noted that premiums increase during the year, provided revenues are higher than $100 per member per month. The excess is used to cover start-up costs and as a reserve for premium rate guarantees extending into the fol-

TABLE 3.4. SURPLUS-DEFICIT DISTRIBUTION METHODOLOGY.

	Industry Trends	Implications
Compensation formulas	No standard methodologies for physician compensation or allocation of surplus or deficit on risk arrangements.	Need to customize methodology to match specific goals and objectives of PHO.
Allocation factors	Trends in physician compensation are away from strictly financial performance measures of utilization and cost. • Most formulas still based largely on productivity factors, but interest is growing in incorporating utilization management and qualitative factors to align financial incentives with managed care priorities. • Estimates are that fewer than 5 percent of all medical groups currently factor utilization management and other quality-of-care measures (patient satisfaction, appropriateness of utilization, citizenship, and patient outcomes) into compensation formulas. • Use of qualitative measures is in evidence only in highly integrated, highly managed group practices.	In initial years, PHO may continue to base most of surplus distribution on measures of financial performance. Over next several years, focus should be on identifying new, more qualitative factors to incorporate into formula. All factors used must be *meaningful, objective, and measurable.* Allocation methodology must be flexible and should change as goals and objectives change and as PHO gains ability to measure different factors.
Measurement tools	Biggest challenge in incorporating new factors is finding appropriate ways to objectively measure them. Many information systems not yet sophisticated enough to capture data and measure performance.	Need to establish appropriate information systems to capture data necessary to measure performance. Important to test integrity of data obtained from managed care organization. Best to reduce relying on managed care organizations to provide all data.
Reserve	Future profit margins will shrink despite improvements in operating performance because of trends toward reducing premium as competition among managed care organizations continues.	Need to establish reserves adequate to cover future losses and be flexible in determining proper withhold levels.
Physician allocation	For a commercial population in a managed care environment, PCP has greatest responsibility and direct control over total care of patient.	Greatest portion of surplus is often allocated to PCP.
Medicare risk	For a Medicare population, specialty care physician use is approximately 2 to 2.5 times that budgeted for commercial use.	Separate risk pool should be established for Medicare risk contracts because of significant variation in population cost and use rates.

TABLE 3.5. POSSIBLE FACTORS FOR SURPLUS ALLOCATION.

Factor	Measurement Tool	Examples
Productivity	Claims data	Gross revenue Net collections Number of patients seen Number of visits per unit of time
Resource/ utilization management	Internally developed targets, HEDIS measures	Average LOS Days/1,000 Specialty visits/1,000 ER visits/1,000 Number of encounters per patient Total cost per patient Average ancillary charge per patient Average total charge per visit Formulary compliance Generic drug utilization Referral patterns Per patient costs for lab, X ray In-network vs. out-of-network use
Patient satisfaction	Patient surveys, work standards, HEDIS measures	Access (e.g., travel, wait for appointment, wait to be seen, time spent with patient, extended hours, PCPs accepting new patients) Patient complaints
Technical quality and outcomes	HEDIS outcomes measures	Percent readmissions Percent repeat surgery Percent deaths following care Percent poisonings Percent patients fully functioning following care Percent cases with adverse reactions Percent immunizations Percent mammographies
Appropriateness of care	Compliance with NCQA and MCAP criteria, peer review	Percent patients treated in inappropriate setting Percent of patients with pre-op days Percent questionable care in short-stay setting Percent C-section rate Percent expense for lack of self-care Percent expense for experimental treatments
Citizenship	Internal targets and work standards	Meeting attendance Coverage Communication Community service
Practice efficiency	Internal standards	Punctuality Ability to keep staff functioning Cost per visit

lowing year.) Out of this premium, $15.68 is retained by the HMO for administration, reinsurance, and contribution to reserves. The reinsurance company is paid $1.66 per member per month (1.66 percent) out of the monthly premium per enrollee.

The remainder is then allocated between a medical services pool and a risk-sharing pool. The medical services pool is the amount of money paid monthly to the physicians medical group for each HMO enrollee. The $47.80 medical services pool capitation rate is paid at the beginning of the month and is the only payment provided for covered services rendered to an enrollee. If the enrollee does not use any medical services during the month, the physicians medical group simply retains the capitation payment. If, on the other hand, the enrollee uses medical services that cost more than the $47.80 capitation, the medical group must absorb the additional cost. Since the catastrophic illness of a single enrollee could have a serious impact on the financial condition of the HMO, an individual stop-loss provision is activated once hospital inpatient services costs for an individual enrollee reach $50,000 during a contract year. The HMO pays for any further in-hospital services from reinsurance proceeds. The medical group must decide to assume all risk for professional medical services (including outside referrals) rather than purchase medical stop-loss insurance.

Through this capitation mechanism, the medical group accepts a significant amount of the risk for providing care to enrollees for a predetermined, prepaid amount. Such an arrangement fosters a financial incentive for the physicians to truly manage the health care of HMO enrollees. The medical group is rewarded for providing preventive medicine and health education, detecting disease in its earliest stages, and providing necessary health care in its most appropriate setting.

Shared-Risk Pool. The mechanism by which the nonphysician risk-sharing arrangement is accomplished is the shared-risk pool. Monthly, $35.67 is allocated to this pool for each HMO enrollee. From this pool, claims for hospital services, prescription drugs (if included), and other covered medical services not encompassed in the medical group's capitation are paid by the HMO. If at the end of a given year, a surplus exists in the shared-risk pool, the HMO pays to the medical group up to 15 percent of the surplus amount over the allocation to the pool during the year to pay for covered services. If, on the other hand, there is a deficit in the shared-risk pool, the medical group must pay the HMO up to 15 percent of the deficit developed in the pool. Again, the $50,000 stop-loss provision is included in this arrangement, so that the medical group and HMO are not financially jeopardized by a single catastrophic illness.

Incentives. The risk-sharing arrangements established between the HMO and physicians medical group do, in fact, afford real economic incentives for the physicians to provide or arrange for cost-effective health care for their patients. At the same time, they do not place the group in financial jeopardy. The risk-sharing arrangements also significantly enhance the potential for the HMO to become a financially secure organization. Although critics may suggest that such financial incentives can have a negative impact on the quality of care, quality is nonetheless guaranteed since the physicians must also participate in quality assurance programs and member complaint and grievance procedures. In addition, the physicians recognize that if enrollees perceive that they are receiving poor-quality health care, they will drop out of the program and choose another health plan offered by the employer. Not only would the physicians' reputations and ability to attract HMO enrollees be threatened but there could also be a negative impact on their fee-for-service business.

As depicted in Figure 3.5, the HMO receives from employers approximately $100 per month per enrolled employee and dependent, to cover all operating expenses. Out of this premium, $20 is retained by the HMO for administration, reserves and profit. The remaining $80 (80 percent of premium) is then actuarially converted into a discounted fee-for-service schedule, with a 10 percent withhold to pay the group physicians and to create a periodic interim payment (PIP) per diem for the hospital. This capitation process actuarially reviews the benefits covered under the premium; the age-and-sex mix of the enrollees, and the projected cost of providing various units of benefit service. This analysis actuarially converts to a utilization budget for the year.

The group or hospital may wish to purchase stop-loss insurance from the HMO to limit its risk. This cost is deducted from the $80 per member per month revenue pool.

If at the end of the performance year the physicians meet their utilization target, the fee-for-service payments have not exceeded the capitation budget and the excess monies are given to the physicians (55 percent PCPs and 45 percent specialists). If the utilization targets are exceeded, the physician withholds (10 percent) are forfeited in amounts up to the level of the deficit. The forfeitures are also shared 55 percent by PCPs and 45 percent by specialists.

In regard to the inpatient hospital activity, it is assumed that PIP is set at $1,200 per day. If utilization is set at 300 days per thousand enrollees and actual utilization is 350 days per thousand enrollees, the actual payment may be $1,000 per day. Under this scenario, the physician withholds are paid to the hospital in the amount equal to the $200 difference between interim and final per diem. In this instance, 55 percent of the withholds come from the specialists and 45 percent from PCPs. If the total withholds do not offset the hospital loss (even with application of inpatient stop-loss insurance), the difference is absorbed by the hospital. If actual utilization is 250 days per thousand enrollees, then the actual payment may be $1,400 per day. In this instance, the hospital gives the physician group practice 50 percent of the excess funds, which are distributed 55 percent to specialists and 45 percent to PCPs.

Figure 3.6 depicts a situation in which the HMO has struck an agreement with an integrated delivery system (shown as "provider organization") in the model. In the model, the HMO receives from employers approximately $93 per month per enrolled employee and dependent to cover all operating expenses. Out of the premium, $14 is retained by the HMO for administration, reserves, and profit.

The remaining 85 percent of premium (or approximately $79) is actuarially converted into a capitation budget (see detailed example, Table 3.3) that is used to reimburse the hospital and PCPs on a capitated per member per month basis. As can be seen in Table 3.3, the results of an actuarial exercise reviewing benefits that are covered under the premium, the age-and-sex mix of the enrollees within the product is analyzed and a projected cost of providing various units of benefit service is calculated. This analysis is actuarially converted to a utilization budget for the performance. The budget is represented in the column titled "Frequency unit/1000" in Table 3.3. This utilization projection multiplied by the average cost per unit for each category of service divided by total member months results in the per member per month capitation shown in the last column of Table 3.3.

The HMO may choose to capitate payments to specialists (their capitation rates are a component of many of the services listed in Table 3.3). As an alternative, the HMO may work to reimburse specialists based upon product or specific procedure.

The provider organization may wish to purchase stop-loss insurance from the HMO to limit its risk. This premium cost would be deducted from the $79 per member per month revenue pool.

In this model, surplus-deficit sharing resides with the provider unit. The physicians and hospital predetermine the distribution of surplus and loss. Based upon the utilization experience during the performance year, the provider unit either distributes a surplus or funds a deficit. In surplus years, they may wish to consider a policy of retaining a portion of the surplus (retained earnings) so as to offset deficit years.

CHAPTER FOUR

NEGOTIATING THE CONTRACT

The essential elements of negotiating a risk contract include understanding the payor's objectives and the provider's limitations, identifying all pertinent issues, performing a financial analysis, and preparing an executive notebook on each payor. Negotiating pointers are designed to help providers reach needed compromises with payors.

Negotiating, Step by Step

Much of your work in preparing for contract negotiations has already been completed as you developed your contracting strategy. The most important steps of a successful negotiation are described in this chapter.

Understand the Payor's Objectives and Limitations

A payor's marketing plan in a given geographic region is generally account-driven. If you can identify the plan's target accounts, perhaps you can assist the payor in (or, in some cases, prevent it from) obtaining accounts. Perhaps your physician group or hospital is a target account.

You should also learn what hospital-physician group contract alternatives are available to the payor to assess your relative leverage in the negotiation. To understand your position with this payor completely, get to know your competition in terms of the issues that are most important to them. For example, what are their comparative product lines? How do their rates compare to yours? Refer back to Exhibit 1.2 for a list of data to be collected about your competitors.

The payor often comes to the table with a specific payment methodology in mind along with a proposed set of payment figures. The payor surely seeks a competitive discount and may offer a fixed payment per day, per case, or per procedure. More and more frequently, plans also want to share risk with providers.

Finally, payors often require uniform administrative policies among their contracted providers. You should understand the policies specific to the payor.

The payor also does its homework about you to understand your strengths, weaknesses, distinctive competencies, and competitive position in the market. Remember that most of the information so gleaned is from publicly available information, which may be somewhat limited. It is therefore critical that you have a keen understanding of your own qualities. What are your niche products? What is your cost structure, and how does it compare to others'? What do you have to offer that is attractive to the plan?

Gather Information About the Payor

Refer back to Exhibit 1.4 for a list of data to be collected about managed care organizations. To supplement the data, follow the checklist in Exhibit 1.3 to analyze the payor's strengths, as well as to identify the benefits of potential affiliation with that organization.

Information may also be gathered informally through conversation with key individuals involved with or knowledgeable about the payor. For example, you could talk to others who deal with the payor, or to employees of the plan. Another tactic might be to have your specialists mix with the payor's specialists. The best conversational techniques to use to gather valuable information are to ask open-ended questions, repeat statements as questions, elicit responses, and request restatement for clarification.

Finally, gain an understanding of the payor's track record in other contracting relationships. Is it able to deliver on promises?

Understand Your Limitations

Assess your ability to accommodate specific accounts brought by the managed care organization. Do you have the capacity and unique service requirements to handle the additional business? Identify your minimum acceptable terms up front. This is dictated by your tolerance for risk as measured against the benefits of gaining a contract with this managed care plan. As you approach the actual negotiation, be realistic about your resources and your time to perform the required analysis.

Perform Financial Analyses

The degree of complexity involved in analyzing the financial ramifications of a contract depends on the type of payment arrangement offered. At a minimum, you should determine the profitability of the contract by comparing estimated revenue to your costs for the mix of volume expected from this contract. The value of the contract may depend on the total volume the plan is able to supply. You may be able to negotiate a deal with prices that vary depending on actual volume. Finally, it is important to take into account the effect of the contract on existing and new business.

Identify All Issues

Once all information has been gathered and analysis performed, you should step back from the detail to identify and prioritize all the issues that are to be raised during the negotiation.

Prepare an Executive Briefing Notebook

An executive briefing notebook is unique to a specific contract and can be used by your designated negotiator(s) to prepare for and conduct the actual negotiation. The notebook should summarize all information developed during the planning stage. All critical issues should be clearly identified, prioritized, and supported by a well-thought-out position. Nonnegotiable items should be separated from those that are negotiable. Issues that are unimportant to the organization should be simply listed as items that require no debate during the actual negotiation. On those issues that are negotiable, the briefing notebook should indicate fallback positions in the event that your opponent does not agree to your first proposal. To ensure that all key terms and issues are addressed during the negotiation, consider using a contract negotiation checklist such as the one shown in Exhibit 4.1.

Seating at the Negotiation

At the actual negotiation, seat positioning can be very important. Nonverbal cues and body language can provide additional valuable information as to which issues appear to be of most importance to the plan, when plan representatives may be bluffing, and how they are reacting to things you have said. In a situation where you are negotiating with two people, be sure to find a position from which both can be watched. If you have another person on your team, you should sit apart from him or her so you convey the effect of "speaking with two different voices." If, on the other hand, you have a large group opposing a small group, keep your group together as evidence of power. If the situation is reversed and you have a small group facing a large group from the opposition, intermingle members of your group with theirs as a means of diffusing their power.

Reach for Compromise

A successful negotiation is characterized by both sides feeling a sense of accomplishment and trust that the other side will keep its end of the bargain. Both parties view the other side as fair in their negotiations, and both are likely to be willing to deal with the other again on other issues.

EXHIBIT 4.1. MANAGED CARE
CONTRACT NEGOTIATION CHECKLIST.

	Item	Comment	Status
Parties	Network, contractor, plan name • Carrier, insured, network • Contact • Title • Phone • Address Third-party administrator • Financial class (HMO, PPO, etc.) • Insurance code • Contact • Title • Phone • Address		
Contract period	Effective date Renewal date Ending date Termination notice • w/c days 30/45/60 • wo/c days 30/45/60		
Services	Services included Excluded		

(Continued)

EXHIBIT 4.1. Continued.

Item	Comment	Status
Contracted reimbursement		
• Excluded services		
• New services		
• Professional services		
• Postdischarge care, transfers		
Continuation of services after contract (applicable or not applicable)		
Services to termination date only		
Full charge after contract expiration		
Remain same		
Split patient's bill		
Other _____		
Amendments allowed (statement provided or not provided)		
Service exclusions (list)		

Item		Comment	Status
Rates	Per diem		
	Percentage of charges		
	Capitation		
	Per case		
	Global per diem:	_____$	
	Per diem:	_____$	
	Other_____		
	Medical or surgical		
	ICU		
	CCU		
	CV surgery		
	Obstetrics		
	C-section		
	Boarder baby		
	Neonatal ICU		
	Peds		
	DOU		
	Adult day care		
	Psych		
	Chemical dependency		
	Rehab		
	Telemetry		
	Skilled nursing		
	Percentage of charges (yes or no):		
	• Inpatient		
	• Ancillary		
	• Outpatient		
	• Stop-loss		
	• Timing for stop-loss		
	• Single admission		
	• Calendar year	$_____	
	• Contract year	$_____	
	• Any 12 consecutive months	$_____	

Item	Comment	Status

Rate changes

Renewal date
Change stated (yes or no)
• ___ days prior to contract
  ending date
Renegotiation required
  (yes or no)
Renegotiation notification
  (yes or n/a)
• Rate increases
• No increase
• Percentage increases   _____ percent
• Price index   _____ percent
Automatic renewal (yes or no)
Allow for amendments
  (yes or no)

Financial incentives

Stop-loss (yes or no)
Channeling exclusivity
  (yes or no)
Volume threshold pricing
  (yes or no)
• Interim rate
• Payback mechanism

Billing and claims processing (check for language)

Eligibility verification by payor
No limit to bill payor
  retrospectively
Coordination of benefits
Exclude payment-in-full
Primary
Secondary
• Up to usual or customary
  charges
• Up to contract terms
Signatories benefit only from
  term of contract
Billing period
Interim billing
Assignment of benefits not
  required
Arbitration process for bill (UR)
  disputes
Right to bill and collect
  coinsurance, deductible,
  and excluded services
30/60/other day limit ____ days

(Continued)

EXHIBIT 4.1. Continued.

Item		Comment	Status

Payments (language or no language)	Exclude language of secondary payor status and limit of payment to contract		
	Identification of coinsurance and deductibles on remittance advice		
	Timing of payment		
	• ____days		
	• Based upon the day hospital receives payment		
	If late payment		
	• Penalty _____; interest rate penalty _____ percent		
	• Hospital can bill beneficiary		
Utilization and retroactive reviews (language or no language)	Third-party bill audits		
	Dispute resolution terms		
	Retrospective reviews		
	If retrospective denials		
Utilization review	Own UR organization (yes or no)		
	Delegated UR (yes or no)		
	Third-party review organization (yes or no)		
	• Contact		
	• Title		
	• Phone		
	• Address		
	Types of UR performed (language or no language)		
	• Preadmission		
	• Concurrent		
	• Retrospective		
	• Extension process		
	• Discharge planning		
	Onsite review		
	• Inspection of medical records and claims		
	• Release of utilization data		
	• Physician contact		

Other considerations (language or no language)	Physician relations
	• Medical staff
	• Bylaws and privileges
	Hospital and payor
	    documentation requirements
	    specified in contract
	Antitrust
	Hospital reputation
	• Directory listing
	• Other uses permitted
	Insurance
	Severability
	Unforeseen circumstances
	Licensing and accreditation

CHAPTER FIVE

SAMPLE HOSPITAL CONTRACT

A sample hospital contract is provided in this chapter to define all the key sections of a managed care agreement. Throughout the sample contract you will find commentary (in italics and bracketed) intended to direct attention to important contract issues.

Once an arrangement between the hospital and a managed care organization has been fully negotiated, the agreement between the parties must be formalized in a legal contract. Most often, the managed care organization drafts the contract and presents it to the hospital for review, although in some circumstances the provider may engage legal counsel to draft the contract. The contract between the payor and the provider generally addresses the obligations of the parties, covered services, payment terms, utilization control, competitive practices, and reporting requirements.

The contract negotiation checklist in Exhibit 4.1 may be helpful in the review process. The draft contract in this chapter is intended to reflect typical provisions; it is not drafted as a preferred model for a hospital.

When reviewing the draft contract, be sure to involve all individuals whose area of responsibility are affected by the terms of the contract. These are likely to be the same individuals identified and included in developing your contracting strategy.

Preliminary Considerations

Under most circumstances, the MCO gives its prospective provider a generic hospital, physician, IPA, or network agreement. There is no ideal contract or contract form. Contract terms vary depending on the particular issues of concern and objectives of each party, the relative bargaining power of each party, and the desired degree of formality. If, for example, a new MCO is very interested in entering a provider's marketplace, the provider may have more leverage. Conversely, a well-established MCO may have its own history with respect to financial, operational, and environmental flexibility. Finally, certain provisions may not be negotiable because of state or federal law.

The contract should also be analyzed to determine which products are included. Is it HMO only? PPO only? Point of service? Multioption? In addition, the applicability of the relationship to noncommercial enrollees, such as Medicare, Medicaid, CHAMPUS, self-insured employers, and others, should also be understood.

Sample Hospital Agreement

PART I. INTRODUCTION
Health Maintenance Organization
Agreement Between

_____

and
_____ Hospital

THIS AGREEMENT is made and entered into on the date set forth on the signature page hereto, by and between _____
(the "Hospital"), a facility duly licensed under the laws of the State of
_____ and located at _____, and
_____ (the "HMO"), a corporation organized under the
_____ laws of the State of _____ and
located at _____.

WHEREAS, HMO provides a plan of health care benefits (the "Plan") to individuals and their eligible family members and dependents who contract with HMO or who are the beneficiaries of a contract with HMO for such benefits ("Members"), and in connection with such Plan, arranges for the provision of health care services, including Hospital Services, to such Members; and

WHEREAS, the Hospital desires to provide Hospital Services to Members in accordance with the terms and conditions of this Agreement as hereinafter set forth; and

WHEREAS, HMO desires to arrange for the services of the Hospital for the benefit of the Members of the Plan.

NOW, THEREFORE, in consideration of the foregoing recitals and the mutual covenants and promises herein contained and other good and valuable consideration, the receipt and sufficiency of which are hereby acknowledged, the parties hereto agree and covenant as follows:

[Generally, the introductory paragraph of the contract identifies the parties and the effective date of the relationship. Although recitals often regard the general description of the nature of the intended relationship between the two parties and are not usually an enforceable part of the contract, they may be considered by an arbitrator or court with respect to the parties' intentions in the event of a dispute.]

PART II. DEFINITIONS

[Although definitions of certain key terms may be scattered throughout the agreement, it is frequently the case, and indeed most helpful, to have them centralized. When reading the contract for the first time, it is important to read the definitions twice: all of them initially, and then a particular term each time it is encountered in its context.]

A. *Covered Services* means those health services and benefits to which Members are entitled under the terms of the applicable Health Maintenance Certificate, which may be amended by HMO from time to time.

[These are the health services and benefits to which members are entitled; they are set forth in a member's evidence of coverage. The scope of covered services should be set forth in a contract. If those services can be changed, the agreement should specify under what circumstances, and with what notice. Noncovered or excluded services should be clearly specified.

Procedures and responsibilities for informing patients of noncovered services generally are also mentioned. For capitated contracts where the hospital is responsible for care provided by other institutions or the physician is responsible for care rendered by specialists, the contract usually indicates the approval process for these services and how any disputes are to be resolved.

In addition, assuming that experimental procedures are excluded from coverage, the standard that the payor uses to define experimental (for example, FDA approval, frequent community usage, etc.) should be specified.

If the third-party payor offers different coverage plans to various enrollee groups, the contract should require the payor to deliver summaries of each document to the provider. Also, for ease of review, reference, and possible future modification, the provider might request that a comprehensive listing of covered services be presented in an exhibit to the contract.]

59

B. *Emergency Services* means those Medically Necessary services provided in connection with an "Emergency," defined as a sudden or unexpected onset of a condition requiring medical or surgical care that the Member receives after the onset of such condition (or as soon thereafter as care can be made available but not more than twenty-four [24] hours after onset) and in the absence of such care the Member could reasonably be expected to suffer serious physical impairment or death. Heart attack, severe chest pain, cardiovascular accident, hemorrhaging, poisoning, major burn, loss of consciousness, serious breathing difficulty, spinal injury, shock, and other acute conditions as a reasonable or prudent person would determine are Emergencies.

[Ideally, the hospital rather than the plan makes the onsite determination as to whether emergency services were rendered, although in either instance the reasonable-layperson standard is being applied to determination of emergency. Additionally, since the Consolidated Omnibus Reconciliation Act of 1986 (COBRA) antidumping provisions require the hospital to screen all patients presenting at the emergency room, the agreement should provide that the plan will pay for such screening services provided to covered persons, regardless of whether or not the patient is ultimately provided emergency services.]

C. *Health Maintenance Certificate* means a contract issued by an HMO to a Member or an employer of Members, specifying the services and benefits available under the HMO's prepaid health benefits program.

D. *Hospital Services* means all inpatient services, emergency room, and outpatient Hospital services that are Covered Services.

E. *Medical Director* means a Physician designated by HMO to monitor and review the provision of Covered Services to Members.

F. *Medically Necessary* services and/or supplies means the use of services or supplies as provided by a Hospital, skilled nursing facility, Physician, or other provider required to identify or treat a Member's illness or injury and which, as determined by HMO's Medical Director or its utilization management committee, are: (1) consistent with the symptoms or diagnosis and treatment of the Member's condition, disease, ailment, or injury; (2) appropriate with regard to standards of good medical practice; (3) not solely for the convenience of the Member, his or her Physician, Hospital, or other health care provider; and (4) the most appropriate supply or level of service that can be safely provided to the Member. When specifically applied to an inpatient Member, it further means that the Member's medical symptoms or condition requires that the diagnosis or treatment cannot be safely provided to the Member as an outpatient.

[Usually, the contract provides that the payor only pays for medically necessary services. This term should be defined as specifically as possible *to inform the hospital as to which services*

payment may be allowed. It is also critical to identify the ultimate decision maker regarding such medical necessity.

The hospital should identify the key decision maker in the first instance. If the payor is to make the decision, then the hospital should be able to have a determination reviewed by either a neutral third party or a committee of provider and payor representatives.]

G. *Member* means both an HMO subscriber and his or her enrolled family members for whom premium payment has been made.

[The contract should define what is meant by member, or covered enrollee. The contract should explain how to determine eligibility and assign responsibility for payment if services are rendered to a noncovered individual.]

H. *Participating Physician* means a Physician who, at the time of providing or authorizing services to a Member, has contracted with or on whose behalf a contract has been entered into with an HMO to provide professional services to Members.
I. *Participating Provider* means a Physician, Hospital, skilled nursing facility, home health agency, or any other duly licensed institution or health professional under contract with the HMO to provide health care services to Members. A list of Participating Providers and their locations is available to each Member upon enrollment. Such a list shall be revised from time to time as the HMO deems necessary.

[The question of defining the participating provider may go hand in hand with identifying the party or parties to the contract. For example, if the provider is part of a larger network, the other facilities should be identified. Likewise, if nonsystem physicians are providing services, they too should be identified and a list of participating providers kept current.]

J. *Physician* means a duly licensed doctor of medicine or osteopathy.
K. *Primary Care Physician* means a Participating Physician who provides primary care services to Members (e.g., general or family practitioner, internist, pediatrician, or such other physician specialty as may be designated by the HMO) and is responsible for referrals of Members to referral Physicians, other Participating Providers, and if necessary, non-Participating Providers.

PART III. HOSPITAL OBLIGATIONS
A. *Covered Services* The Hospital shall provide to Members those Hospital Services that the Hospital has the capacity to provide. Such services shall be provided by the Hospital in accordance with the provisions of its Articles of

Incorporation and Bylaws and medical staff Bylaws and the appropriate terms of this Agreement.

[The provider organization agrees to provide or arrange for provision of hospital services as part of the previously defined covered services. It is important to determine whether this is to include affiliated entities, such as nursing homes, laboratories, and outpatient service organizations, as well as hospital-based physician services such as pathology, anesthesia, or radiology.]

B. *Standards of Care* Hospital shall render Hospital Services to Members in an economical and efficient manner consistent with professional standards of medical care generally accepted in the medical community. Hospital shall not discriminate in the treatment of Members and, except as otherwise required by this Agreement, shall make its services available to Members in the same manner as to its other patients. In the event that an admission of a Member cannot be accommodated by the Hospital, the Hospital shall make the same efforts to arrange for the provision of services at another facility approved by the HMO that it would make for other patients in similar circumstances. In the event that the Hospital shall provide Member non-Covered Services, the Hospital shall, prior to the provision of such non-Covered Services, inform the Member:

1. Of the service(s) to be provided,
2. That HMO will not pay for or be liable for said services, and
3. That the Member will be financially liable for such services.

[A contract may include various other "standard of care" requirements. Some of the more common are

1. Hold Harmless. The state and federal Health Care Financing Administration require that the provider agree not to bill a member except for deductibles, copayments and noncovered services. Because this requirement and the specific language are often dictated by state law, there is rarely any negotiating of these provisions.

2. Nondiscrimination. A clause may also be included to prohibit other types of discrimination, on the basis of race, color, sex, age, religion, and national origin. The provider is likely to be required to agree not to treat a particular payor's beneficiaries any differently than it treats all other patients.

3. Participation in UR/QA (Utilization Review or Quality Assurance) Activity. Most managed care contracts require the provider to comply with the payor's utilization review program and quality assurance program. The programs should be clearly and separately defined in the contract. Are there preauthorization or preadmission certification requirements? If so, how is coverage verified? Generally, eligibility verification may occur through presentation of identification cards or telephone verification of eligibility. It is possible that the managed care organization accepts the hospital's existing UR/QA program. The program should further specify whether concurrent review and retrospective review is part of the UR/QA program.

The provider should be able to obtain from the payor updated and detailed information and data no less than quarterly, preferably monthly, regarding utilization.

Finally, the mechanism for appealing a utilization decision should be set forth. Those appeal rights may depend on how the initial review is conducted. If a determination is made solely by the payor (for example, by the payor's medical director), a review including other providers or neutral reviews may be appropriate. The standard of review (whether it is a review of medical necessity or simply of the reasonableness of the original decision) should be specified and understood. If the appeal is to be conducted by a group, the members of that group and their qualifications and specialties should be consistent with the particular issue being appealed.]

C. *Member Identification* Except in an Emergency, the Hospital shall provide the Hospital Inpatient Services to a Member only when the Hospital has received certification from HMO in advance of admission of such Member. Services that have not been so approved or authorized shall be the sole financial responsibility of the Hospital.

[At the time of preauthorization for an admission, the payor should establish a recommended length of stay. The process for extending the admission beyond the recommended stay should be clearly set forth.

It should be noted that a provider may be held liable if it discharges a patient in accordance with the length of stay authorized by the payor but prior to a determination by the provider of the medical appropriateness of that discharge. Thus, a provider may not rely on the payor's decision and retains ultimate responsibility for patient care notwithstanding reimbursement decisions.]

If, and to the extent that, the Hospital is not authorized to perform preadmission testing, the Hospital agrees to accept the results of qualified and timely laboratory, radiological, and other tests and procedures that may be performed on a Member prior to admission. The Hospital will not require that duplicate tests or procedures be performed after the Enrollee is admitted, unless such tests and procedures are Medically Necessary.

In an Emergency, the Hospital shall immediately proceed to render Medically Necessary services to the Member. The Hospital shall also contact the HMO within twenty-four (24) hours of the emergency treatment visit or Emergency Admission. The HMO has twenty-four (24) hour on-call nurse coverage for notification of Emergency Services or admissions.

[The hospital should not be required to verify eligibility or seek preauthorization in the event of an emergency.]

If the Hospital fails to notify the HMO within the required time period, neither the HMO nor the Member shall be liable for charges for Hospital Services rendered subsequent to the required notification period that are deemed by HMO not to be Medically Necessary.

The Hospital shall cooperate with and abide by the HMO's programs that monitor and evaluate whether Hospital services provided to Members in accordance with this Agreement are Medically Necessary and consistent with professional standards of medical care generally accepted in the medical community. Such programs include, but are not limited to, utilization management, quality assurance review, and grievance procedures. In connection with the HMO's programs, the Hospital shall permit the HMO's utilization management personnel to visit Members in the Hospital and, to the extent permitted by applicable laws, to inspect and copy health records (including medical records) of Members maintained by the Hospital for the purposes of concurrent and retrospective utilization management, discharge planning, and other program management purposes.

The Hospital shall cooperate with the HMO in complying with applicable laws relating to the HMO.

PART IV. LICENSURE AND ACCREDITATIONS

The Hospital represents that it is duly licensed by the Department of Health of the State of _____ to operate a Hospital, is a qualified provider under the Medicare program, and is accredited by the Joint Commission on the Accreditation of Healthcare Organizations ("Joint Commission"). The Hospital shall maintain in good standing such license and accreditation and shall notify the HMO immediately should any action of any kind be initiated against the Hospital which could result in:

1. The suspension or loss of such license;
2. The suspension or loss of such accreditation; or
3. The imposition of any sanctions against the Hospital under the Medicare or Medicaid programs.

The Hospital shall furnish to the HMO such evidence of licensure, Medicare qualification, and accreditation as the HMO may request.

PART V. RECORDS

A. The Hospital shall maintain with respect to each Member receiving Hospital Services pursuant to this Agreement a standard Hospital medical record in such form, containing such information, and preserved for such time period(s) as are required by the rules and regulations of the _____ Department of Health, the Medicare program, and the Joint Commission. The original Hospital medical records shall be and remain the property of the Hospital and shall not be removed or transferred from the Hospital except in accordance with applicable laws and general Hospital policies, rules, and regulations relating thereto; provided, however, that the HMO shall have the right, in accordance with paragraph (B) below, to inspect, review, and make copies of such records upon request. B. Upon consent of the Member and a request for such records or information, the Hospital shall provide copies of information contained in the medical records of Members to other authorized providers of health care services and to the HMO for the purpose of facilitating the delivery of appropriate health care services to Members and carrying out the purposes and provisions of this Agreement, and shall facilitate the sharing of such records among health care providers involved in a Member's care. The HMO and, if required, authorized state and federal agencies shall have the right upon request to inspect at reasonable times and in a manner that does not interfere with the normal business operations of the Hospital and to obtain copies of all records that are maintained by the Hospital relating to the care of Members pursuant to this Agreement. The HMO represents and warrants that it has obtained any and all Member releases with respect to said medical records. The HMO shall pay Hospital _____ per page for any copies of records so requested.

[The payor usually requires that the provider allow access to or copies of medical and financial records to verify coverage and payment. If access is to be accomplished through an onsite inspection, the payor should be required to do so in a manner that does not interfere with the normal business operations of the provider. Similarly, the payor should be required to reimburse the provider for reasonable copying costs of any records. For example, stating a specific cost per page or pegging it to the Medicare copying rate may avoid any question about the costs in the future. Often providers are required to provide information to the state or the federal government as may be necessary for the payor to comply with state and federal laws.

The managed care organization should be required to provide detailed reports on utilization and quality. These should be correlated with financial reports, to the extent feasible and appropriate.

If the contract calls for release of patient-specific information by the provider, it is important to consider the requirements of state laws regarding confidentiality and prior patient authorization. The provider should also seek indemnification by the payor for any improper release of patient information that the payor obtains from the provider. The managed care organization should be the party responsible for obtaining a patient's release to review those medical records. Generally, those releases are contained as part of the enrollee application. Within the contract, the payor should represent and warrant that it has obtained any and all necessary member consents.

If the payor has not detailed a release with respect to certain protected categories of medical records, such as HIV or mental health and substance abuse, it may be appropriate for the hospital to make a good-faith attempt to obtain a patient's release for those records. The hospital cannot, however, guarantee that it will be able to obtain a patient's consent with respect to any records, and payment should not be denied if it is unable to obtain a patient's consent to release those records to the payor for purposes of utilization review or quality assurance.]

PART VI. INSURANCE AND INDEMNIFICATION

A. *Insurance* The Hospital shall secure and maintain at its expense throughout the term of this Agreement such policy or policies of general liability and professional liability insurance in amounts of $_____/$_____ annual aggregate to insure the Hospital, its agents, and employees against any claim or claims for damages arising by reason of injury or death, occasioned directly or indirectly by the performance or nonperformance of any service by the Hospital, its agents, or employees. Upon request, the Hospital shall provide the HMO with a copy of the policy (or policies) or certificate(s) of insurance that evidence compliance with the foregoing insurance requirements.

[Acceptable limits of coverage should be explicitly set forth in the contract.]

B. *Indemnification* The Hospital and HMO each shall indemnify and hold the other harmless from any and all liability, loss, damage, claim, or expense of any kind, including costs and attorney's fees, arising out of the performance of this Agreement and for which the other is solely responsible.

[The purpose of indemnification clauses is to require that each respective party bear the burden of any claims arising from their respective conduct. The hospital should not enter into any contract in which it is indemnifying the payor but the payor does not indemnify the hospital. Thus, if indemnification provisions are included at all, they should be reciprocal. One consideration with respect to indemnification provisions is whether any such indemnity is outside the scope of the hospital's insurance coverage. Often, professional liability insurance policies exclude coverage for claims incurred by contract, such as through indemnification provisions with managed care organizations. Thus, any such provision should be qualified to limit indemnification to the extent of professional and general liability insurance coverage.]

PART VII. MEDICAL STAFF MEMBERSHIP

Notwithstanding any other provision of this Agreement, a Participating Physician may not admit or treat a Member in the Hospital unless he or she is a member in good standing of the Hospital's organized medical staff with appropriate clinical privileges to admit and treat such a Member.

PART VIII. MANAGED CARE ORGANIZATION OBLIGATIONS

A. The HMO shall provide to or for the benefit of each Member an identification card, which shall be presented for purposes of assisting the Hospital in verifying Member eligibility. In addition, the HMO shall maintain other verification procedures by which the Hospital may confirm the eligibility of any Member.

[The payor should provide verification of coverage and notify the hospital with respect to enrollments and disenrollments. The process for verification of coverage should be clearly understood and operationally compatible with the hospital's systems. Usually, the payor is responsible for providing appropriate identification cards to all enrollees. Since, however, benefits may vary from plan to plan and enrollee to enrollee, the identification card should, at a minimum, indicate how to verify benefits and member eligibility with a telephone call and indicate where to send billing statements.

The contract should specify who bears the risk of retroactive terminations. Some contracts provide that if an enrollee is retroactively terminated although the provider verified coverage at the time services were rendered, the provider is nevertheless liable for billing the enrollee and attempting to collect directly from the enrollee for those services. Some managed care organizations are willing to share the burden of retroactive termination that may arise when the employer or group is delinquent in informing the managed care organization of employee terminations.

For example, if an individual to whom service has been provided turns out to have been ineligible on the dates services were rendered, the provider may attempt to collect directly from the patient for three regular billing cycles. If it remains unable to collect from the patient for those services, the managed care organization then bears the burden of payment.

If possible, the contract should provide that the payor guarantees payment to the provider for services rendered in reliance on the payor's eligibility verification process.]

B. The HMO shall provide thirty (30) days' advance notice to the Hospital of any changes in Covered Services or in the copayments or conditions of coverage applicable thereto.

[The need to keep a constant definition of covered services is especially critical in a capitated contract. If, for example, a new benefit is mandated by the state, the provider should have the ability to renegotiate and adjust the capitation payment to account for any additional costs of covering that benefit.]

C. The HMO will, whenever an individual, admitted or referred, is not a Member, advise the Hospital within thirty (30) days from the date of receipt of an invoice from the Hospital for services to such an individual. In such cases, the Hospital shall directly bill the individual or another third party payor for services rendered to such individual.

[As discussed above, the HMO may not have current eligibility information if the employer was delinquent in informing the HMO of employee terminations.]

D. In the event continued stay or services are denied after a patient has been admitted, the HMO or its representative shall inform the patient that services have been denied.

[Sometimes this burden falls to the hospital.

Other common managed care organization obligations include:

1. Timely Payment. One of the advantages of contracting with a managed care plan may be prompt payment for services. Often, the contract creates incentives to ensure prompt payment. For example, interest may be charged if payment is not made within a specified number of days following billing. Some contracts also grant the provider the right to cancel a contract if timely payment is not made.

2. Marketing. The managed care organization is obliged to enroll members and market the contracting provider to employers and other potential enrollees in the community. If possible, it may be appropriate and desirable to set certain agreed-upon marketing projections.

3. Exclusivity. Some contracts contain one-way exclusivity clauses that prohibit providers from signing contracts with other managed care organizations. Such clauses limit a provider's ability to take advantage of new market opportunities and may prove quite burdensome. Since these provisions serve to benefit only the payor, it is generally wise for providers to avoid them. On the other hand, providers may be able to negotiate that certain other hospitals or physician groups be excluded from the payor's network as a means of maintaining market share.

4. "Most Favored Nation" Clauses. The contract may contain a nondiscriminatory pricing clause that prohibits the provider from offering another payor more favorable prices. This type of restriction can cause problems when the provider is considering a contract with another managed care plan that is offering more market share or other benefits in exchange for the favorable payment arrangement. If such a clause is required, it should be written in such a way that the payor is subject to the same restrictions as other payors. As an example, before qualifying for a greater discount, the original payor would have to guarantee the same volume as that promised by the new payor. Hospital counsel should review exclusivity or "most favored nation" clauses for antitrust implications based upon the facts and circumstances presented.]

PART IX. USE OF NAME

Except as provided in this paragraph, neither the HMO nor the Hospital shall use the other's name, symbols, trademarks, or service marks in advertising or promotional material or otherwise. The HMO shall have the right to use the name of the Hospital for purposes of marketing, informing Members of the identity of the Hospital, and otherwise to carry out the terms of this Agreement. The

Hospital shall have the right to use the HMO's name in its informational or promotional materials with the HMO's prior approval, which approval shall not be unreasonably withheld.

[It is common to have a provision providing that both parties may use the name of the other in their marketing efforts, so long as the payor's use of the hospital's name is limited to its name, location, and scope of services. Any further use of the hospital name should require the hospital's prior approval.]

PART X. COMPENSATION

The Hospital will be compensated by the HMO for all Medically Necessary Covered Services provided to Members in accordance with the provisions of Attachment A annexed hereto and incorporated herein.

[This section addresses the agreed-upon payment methodology and terms of payment. Payment arrangements will vary by methodology, according to inpatient or outpatient status, by type of service, by product, or by other factors. Specific payment terms are most frequently contained in a separate attachment to the contract because they are more often subject to amendment than other portions of the contract. (Although there is a reference to "Attachment A" in this section, no attachment is provided with the sample contract in this chapter. Chapter Three offered in-depth discussion of payment methodologies and reimbursement terms that would be set forth in a typical "Attachment A.")]

PART XI. PAYMENT TO THE HOSPITAL BY THE HMO

For Hospital Services rendered to Members, the Hospital shall invoice the HMO. Except for the Hospital Services that the HMO determines require further review under the HMO's utilization management procedures, or except when there are circumstances beyond the control of the HMO, including submission of incomplete claims, the HMO shall make payment of invoices for Hospital Services within thirty (30) calendar days after the HMO's receipt thereof. The HMO authorized copayments shall be collected by the Hospital from the Member, and the Member shall be solely responsible for the payment of such copayments. All billings by the Hospital shall be considered final unless adjustments are requested in writing by the Hospital within sixty (60) days after the date of discharge of the Member or date of service, whichever occurs later. The Hospital shall interim bill the HMO every thirty (30) days for patients whose length of stay is greater than thirty (30) days.

[The contract indicates how the provider is to notify the payor of services performed (as by means of standard hospital bill, specially designed payor invoice, UB-92, magnetic tape, and the like).

If a hospital, or hospital system, is capitated, no invoice is rendered by the hospital; rather, the burden shifts to the HMO to pay the hospital monthly based upon the HMO's enrollment.

Risk pool settlement terms, such as timing of payment, interest earned on the pool, and interest charges for late payment of the settlement, should also be addressed in the contract. The contract should specify the party responsible for holding the risk pool funds and generally require that all settlements be made through the payor. For example, a hospital holding a risk pool with a surplus may be required to remit all but its share to the plan, which then allocates the remainder among physicians and other affected parties.

The contract also addresses responsibilities for collecting payments from sources other than the payor, and ownership of the revenues. For example, the managed care plan may be responsible for collecting, and entitled to keep payments from, an enrollee's primary insurance (known as "coordination of benefits"). Providers are generally assigned responsibility for collecting patient copayments and deductibles.]

PART XII. PROHIBITIONS ON MEMBER BILLING

The Hospital hereby agrees that in no event, including but not limited to nonpayment by the HMO, the HMO's insolvency, or breach of this Agreement, shall the Hospital bill, charge, collect a deposit from, seek compensation, remuneration or reimbursement from, or have any recourse against a Member or persons other than the HMO acting on a Member's behalf for services provided pursuant to this Agreement. This provision shall not prohibit collection of copayment on the HMO's behalf in accordance with the terms of the Health Maintenance Certificate between the HMO and Member. The Hospital further agrees that:

1. This provision shall survive the termination of this Agreement regardless of the cause giving rise to termination and shall be construed to be for the benefit of the Member; and
2. This provision supersedes any oral or written contrary agreement now existing or hereafter entered into between the Hospital and Member, or persons acting on their behalf.

[As mentioned above, because the precise language of hold-harmless clauses is often dictated by state law, there is rarely any negotiating of these provisions.]

PART XIII. INSPECTION OF RECORDS

Upon request, and at reasonable times, the HMO and the Hospital shall make available to the other for review such books, records, utilization information, and other documents or information relating directly to any determination required by this Agreement. All such information shall be held by the receiving party in confidence and shall only be used in connection with the administration of this Agreement.

[Access to any nonpublic information should go hand in hand with confidentiality provisions.]

PART XIV. COORDINATION OF BENEFITS

The Hospital agrees to cooperate with the HMO toward effective implementation of any provisions of the HMO's Health Maintenance Certificates relating to coordination of benefits and claims by third parties. The Hospital shall forward to the HMO any payments received from a third-party payor for authorized Hospital Services where the HMO has made payment to the Hospital covering such Hospital Services and such third-party payor is determined to be primarily obligated for such Hospital Services under applicable Coordination of Benefits rules. Such payment shall not exceed the amount paid to the Hospital by the HMO. Except as otherwise required by law, the Hospital agrees to permit the HMO to bill and process forms for any third-party payor on Hospital's behalf, or to bill such third party directly, as determined by the HMO. The Hospital further agrees to waive, when requested, any claims against third-party payors for its provision of Hospital Services to Members and to execute any further documents that reasonably may be required or appropriate for this purpose. Any such waiver shall be contingent upon the HMO's payment to the Hospital of its (HMO's) obligations for charges incurred by Member.

PART XV. TERM AND TERMINATION

[The contract should specify what the term is. If it is for a specified term, the renewal process should likewise be identified. For example, if the agreement is for one year, the parties should notify each other no less than sixty days prior to the expiration date of their intent to renew. If the contract is self-renewing (as by stating that it is effective unless and until affirmatively terminated by one of the parties), there should be some mechanism built in for adjusting rates. For example, the contract may state that sixty days prior to each anniversary date of the agreement, the parties shall agree upon any adjustment to financial terms of the agreement for the following year.]

A. This Agreement shall take effect on the effective date set forth on the signature page and shall continue for a period of one year or until terminated as provided herein.

1. Either party may terminate this Agreement without cause upon at least ninety (90) days' written notice prior to the term of this Agreement.

*[Regardless of the term of the contract, it may be terminable upon, for example, ninety (90) days'
notice. Some managed care organizations require that the contract terminate over the course of a
year on a month-by-month basis with respect to enrollees covered by group contracts that expire in
a particular month.]*

2. Either party may terminate this Agreement with cause upon at least thirty
(30) days' prior written notice.

*[If the contract is to terminate with cause (including loss of licenses, loss of insurance, insol-
vency, or bankruptcy), this should be specified. If one cause is for breach of the agreement, it
should be only for a material breach of the agreement and provide for an opportunity to cure the
alleged breach. If termination were for less than a material breach, it would effectively foreshorten
a "no cause" termination period to thirty days.*

*If enrollees have selected physicians as their primary care physicians who are employed
by, or whose assets are owned by, the hospital, the hospital may want to be in control of any
notices that go out to the patients regarding termination of a particular managed care relationship. At a minimum, letters going out to the patients should be reviewed and approved by
both parties.]*

B. The HMO shall have the right to terminate this Agreement immediately by
notice to the Hospital upon the occurrence of any of the following events:

1. The suspension or revocation of the Hospital's license;
2. The suspension, revocation, or loss of the Hospital's Joint Commission accreditation or Medicare qualification; or
3. Breach of Part III(B) (Hospital Standards of Care) or Part XII (Prohibitions
   on Member Billing) of this Agreement.

C. Hospital shall have the right to terminate this Agreement immediately by
notice to the HMO upon the occurrence of any of the following events:

1. The suspension or revocation of the HMO's license;
2. The receivership or other control of the HMO's operations by the State
Commissioner of Insurance.

D. The HMO shall continue to pay the Hospital in accordance with the
provision of Attachment A for Hospital Services provided by the Hospital to
Members hospitalized at the time of termination of this Agreement, pending
clinically appropriate discharge or transfer to an HMO-designated Hospital
when medically appropriate as determined by the HMO. In continuing to

provide such hospital services, the Hospital shall abide by the applicable terms and conditions of this Agreement.

[Often, in managed care contracts, the provider is required to continue to provide services to individuals who are inpatients on the date of termination. This obligation extends to either the date of discharge or the date of transfer to another participating hospital. It would be appropriate to require the payor to reimburse the hospital based on hospital's charges for any such post-termination services, but it is most customary for payment to be based upon the preexisting contractual terms. If the hospital is paid on a capitation basis, any post-termination services should be reimbursed as fee-for-service.

Certain other obligations, such as confidentiality of financial and medical records, access to such records if there is any reconciliation of amounts due or for audit purposes, and any covenant not to compete, remain in effect after the contract otherwise terminates.]

PART XVI. ADMINISTRATION
The Hospital agrees to abide by and cooperate with the HMO administrative policies including, but not limited to, claims procedures, copayment collections, and duplicate coverage/subrogation recoveries. Nothing in this Agreement shall be construed to require the Hospital to violate, breach, or modify its written policies and procedures unless specifically agreed to herein.

PART XVII. MEMBER GRIEVANCES
The Hospital agrees to cooperate in and abide by the HMO grievance procedures in resolving Member's grievances related to the provision of Hospital Services. In this regard, the HMO shall bring to the attention of appropriate Hospital officials all Member complaints involving the Hospital, and the Hospital shall, in accordance with its regular procedure, investigate such complaints and use its best efforts to resolve them in a fair and equitable manner. The Hospital agrees to notify the HMO promptly of any action taken or proposed with respect to the resolution of such complaints and the avoidance of similar complaints in the future. The Hospital shall notify the HMO after it has received a complaint from an HMO Member.

[A provider is often requested to comply with and participate in any grievance proceedings brought by members. The contract should require the payor to notify the hospital promptly upon receipt of any grievance by a member pertaining to the hospital's care. Moreover, the hospital should not merely be allowed to "cooperate" in the process but entitled to be actively involved in any dispute since it may accompany a potential malpractice allegation.]

PART XVIII. MISCELLANEOUS
A. If any term, provision, covenant, or condition of this Agreement is invalid, void, or unenforceable, the rest of the Agreement shall remain in full force and

effect. The invalidity or nonenforceability of any term or provision hereof shall in no way affect the validity or enforceability of any other term or provision.

B. This Agreement contains the complete understanding and agreement between the Hospital and the HMO and supersedes all representations, understandings, or agreements prior to the execution hereof.

[The contract should provide that the underlying agreement and any external documents that are incorporated by reference constitute the entire agreement between the parties.]

C. The HMO and the Hospital agree that, to the extent compatible with the separate and independent management of each, they shall at all times maintain an effective liaison and close cooperation with each other to provide maximum benefits to Members at the most reasonable cost consistent with quality standards of Hospital care.

D. No waiver, alteration, amendment, or modification of this Agreement shall be valid unless in each instance a written memorandum specifically expressing such waiver, alteration, amendment, or modification is made and subscribed by a duly authorized officer of the Hospital and a duly authorized officer of the HMO.

[Generally speaking, amendments to managed care contracts should be made in writing only. Thus, oral agreements with respect to the relationship between the parties would not be valid. If the payor is going to change other documents—such as UR/QA procedures; evidences of coverage that enumerate covered services, policies, or procedures; or other documents, all of which substantially change the financial needs and expectations for the hospital—any such amendments should require notice consistent with termination of the agreement.]

E. Neither party shall assign its rights, duties, or obligations under this Agreement without the express, written permission of the other party.

[The hospital may want to have an agreement that is assignable to its affiliates or subsidiaries. A third-party payor may ask for a reciprocal provision. Often, a payor may further request that the contract be assignable to any purchaser or successor organization. The hospital may not want to allow for such assignment without knowing who the assignee is going to be and determining its financial and operational capabilities.]

F. None of the provisions of this Agreement are intended to create nor shall be deemed to create any relationship between the HMO and the Hospital other than that of independent entities contracting with each other hereunder solely for the purpose of effecting the provisions of this Agreement. Neither of the parties hereto, nor any of their respective employees shall be construed to be the agent, employer, employee, or representative of the other.

[Most contracts contain a provision stating that the managed care plan and the provider have an independent contractual relationship. The purpose of this provision is to refute any presumption that the provider serves as an employee of the health plan. A related clause often used states that nothing in the agreement should be construed to require physicians to recommend a course of treatment that is deemed professionally inappropriate.

This clause is to affirm that the plan does not participate in the practice of medicine.]

G. This Agreement shall be construed in accordance with the laws of the State of _____.

[H. Dispute Resolution The contract may provide for arbitration or other alternative modes of dispute resolution. Any such arbitration provisions or dispute resolution provisions (such as negotiation and mediation) should specify the disputes to be arbitrated, identify the decision maker(s), and describe the process and whether the findings are binding or whether there are further appeal rights. Finally, the parties should allocate responsibility for costs of the mediator or arbitration.]

I. The headings and numbers of sections and paragraphs contained in this Agreement are for reference purposes only and shall not affect in any way the meaning or interpretation of this Agreement.

The provisions of this Agreement shall be sent by registered mail or certified mail, return receipt requested, postage prepaid to:

_____

_____

_____

_____

and to the Hospital at:

_____

_____

_____

_____

[A managed care contract usually specifies where notices should be submitted to the other party and to whose attention such notices should be delivered. The notice provision should allow for notice by overnight delivery services (such as Federal Express) or, if appropriate, facsimile.]

IN WITNESS WHEREOF, the foregoing Agreement between _____ _____ and the Hospital is entered into by and between the undersigned parties, to be effective the _____ day of _____, 19___.

By:

Title: _____

Date: _____

HOSPITAL

By: _____

Title: _____

Date: _____

[The signature page should indicate who is signing the agreement on behalf of the hospital. Clearly, only individuals who are authorized by the organization to enter into such agreements should be allowed to sign.]

CHAPTER SIX

SAMPLE PHYSICIAN CONTRACT

This chapter presents a sample primary care physician agreement with commentary (identified, as in Chapter Five, with italic text in brackets) to define key contract sections and direct attention to important contract issues.

The contracts that managed care organizations most typically present to physicians are standard agreements. Unfortunately, many physicians never read the agreement, much less seek professional review. Although a payor is usually reluctant to change any standard provisions, if the physician is part of a large provider group leverage may be possible, and even in an individual situation secondary documents may amend or clarify the base agreement. Certain provisions may not be negotiable because of state or federal law. A physician should not, simply on the belief that a contract cannot be changed or because colleagues have already signed it, fail to read the agreement or request modifications.

Contracts with specialists are similar to primary care physician agreements but are unlikely to contain gatekeeper or other capitation provisions. Specialists are, though, probably involved with other types of risk sharing and utilization management. The contract negotiation checklist in Exhibit 4.1 may be helpful in the review process.

This draft contract is intended to reflect typical provisions; it is drafted neither as a preferred model for a physician nor as a means of supplanting legal or financial advice.

Sample Physician Agreement

PART I. INTRODUCTION
Agreement Between

_____

and
Primary Care Physician

_____

THIS AGREEMENT is made and entered into on the date set forth on the signature page hereto, by and between _____
Inc., a _____ corporation (hereinafter referred to as "HMO"), which is organized and operated as a health maintenance organization under the laws of the State of _____, and the individual physician or group practice identified on the signature page hereto (hereinafter referred to as "Primary Care Physician").

   WHEREAS, the HMO desires to operate a health maintenance organization pursuant to the laws of the State of _____;

   WHEREAS, the Primary Care Physician is a duly licensed physician (or if Primary Care Physician is a legal entity, the members of such entity are duly licensed physicians) in the State of _____ whose license(s) is (are) without limitation or restriction, and

[Although there is nothing wrong with having a statement here that the primary care physician's license is not restricted, the body of the contract generally contains this language and provides that failure to maintain the license is ground for termination (Section M).]

   WHEREAS, the HMO has as an objective the development and expansion of cost-effective means of delivering quality health services to Members, as defined herein, particularly through prepaid health care plans, and the Primary Care Physician concurs in, actively supports, and will contribute to the achievement of this objective, and

   WHEREAS, the HMO and the Primary Care Physician mutually desire to enter into an Agreement whereby the Primary Care Physician shall provide and coordinate the health care services to Members of the HMO.

   NOW, THEREFORE, in consideration of the premises and mutual covenants herein contained and for good and valuable consideration, it is mutually covenanted and agreed by and between the parties hereto as follows:

[Generally, the introductory paragraph of the contract identifies the parties and the effective date of the relationship. Although recitals often regard the general description of the nature of the intended relationship between the two parties and are not usually an enforceable part of the contract, they may be considered by an arbitrator or court with respect to the parties' intentions in the event of a dispute.]

PART II. DEFINITIONS

[Although definitions of certain key terms may be scattered throughout the agreement, it is frequently the case, and indeed most helpful, to have the definitions centralized. When reading the contract for the first time, it is important to read the definitions twice: all of them initially, and then a particular term each time it is encountered in its context.]

A. *Covered Services* means those health services and benefits to which Members are entitled under the terms of an applicable Evidence of Coverage, which may be amended by the HMO from time to time upon no less than sixty (60) days' prior notice to the Physician.

[This definition notes the HMO's right to revise the covered services to which the member is entitled and for which the primary care physician is compensated. If the physicians are capitated for those services, a mechanism needs to be available to revise the capitation rate accordingly for changed definitions of covered services that expand or contract the scope of services.

In addition, assuming that experimental procedures are excluded from coverage, the standard that the payor uses to define experimental—for example, FDA approval, frequent community usage, etc.—should be specified.

If the third-party payor offers different coverage plans to various enrollee groups, the contract should require the payor to deliver summaries of each document to the provider. Also, for ease of review, reference, and possible future modification, the provider might request that a comprehensive listing of covered services be presented in an exhibit or attachment to the contract.]

B. *Emergency Services* means those Medically Necessary services provided in connection with an "Emergency," defined as a sudden or unexpected onset of a condition requiring medical or surgical care that the Member secures after the onset of such condition or as soon thereafter as care can be made available but in any case not later than twenty-four (24) hours after onset, and in the absence of such care the Member could reasonably be expected to suffer serious physical impairment or death. Heart attack, severe chest pain, cardiovascular accident, hemorrhaging, poisoning, major burn, loss of consciousness, serious breathing difficulty, spinal injury, shock, and other acute conditions as a reasonably prudent person would determine are Emergencies.

[The definition for emergency services should be identical to the definition used in a member's evidence of coverage agreement. The examples are useful in illustrating types of conditions that are considered emergencies. Many states are enacting or considering legislation applying a "reasonable layperson" standard to the determination of emergency.]

   C. *Encounter Form* means a record of services provided by the Physician to Members in a format acceptable to the HMO.

[In stating that the encounter form must be acceptable to the HMO, the contract allows the HMO to change its requirements in the future. The forms most commonly used are the HCFA 1500 or successor forms, even if the physician is reimbursed on a capitation rather than fee-for-service basis.]

   D. *Evidence of Coverage* means a contract issued by the HMO to a Member or an employer of Members specifying the services and benefits available under the HMO's prepaid health benefits program.

   E. *Health Professionals* means doctors of medicine, doctors of osteopathy, dentists, nurses, chiropractors, podiatrists, optometrists, physician assistants, clinical psychologists, social workers, pharmacists, occupational therapists, physical therapists, and other professionals engaged in the delivery of health services who are licensed, practice under an institutional license, and are certified or practice under other authority consistent with the laws of the state of

   _____.

   F. *Medical Director* means a Physician designated by the HMO to monitor and review the provision of Covered Services to Members.

[The medical director may be a representative of the HMO or an IPA.]

   G. *Medically Necessary* services and/or supplies means the use of services or supplies as provided by a Hospital, skilled nursing facility, Physician, or other provider required to identify or treat a Member's illness or injury and which, as determined by the HMO's Medical Director or its utilization review committee, are: (1) consistent with the symptoms or diagnosis and treatment of the Member's condition, disease, ailment, or injury; (2) appropriate with regard to standards of good medical practice; (3) not solely for the convenience of the Member, his or her physician, Hospital, or other health care provider; and (4) the most appropriate supply or level of service that can be safely provided to the Member.

[This clause gives the HMO authority to deny coverage for a medically appropriate procedure where another procedure is also appropriate. Although this clause does not explicitly address the

subject, it is intended to give the HMO the right to cover only the most cost-effective, medically appropriate procedure. An alternative way of addressing the issue is to state specifically as one of the criteria that allowable procedures are performed in the least costly setting or manner appropriate to treat the enrollee's medical condition.]

       When specifically applied to an inpatient Member, it further means that the Member's medical symptoms or condition require that the diagnosis or treatment cannot be safely provided to the Member as an outpatient.

[This last sentence makes clear the preference of outpatient care over inpatient care.]

       H. *Member* means both a Subscriber and his or her eligible family members for whom premium payment has been made.

[Member is usually synonymous with enrollee. The definition of member should be consistent with the definition used in the HMO group or individual enrollment agreement.]

       I. *Participating Physician* means a Physician who, at the time of providing or authorizing services to a Member, has contracted with or on whose behalf a contract has been entered into, e.g., through the physician's membership in a group practice, IPA, or PHO, with the HMO to provide professional services to Members.
       J. *Participating Provider* means a Physician, Hospital, skilled nursing facility, home health agency, or any other duly licensed institution or Health Professional under contract with the HMO to provide professional and Hospital services to Members.
       K. *Physician* means a duly licensed doctor of medicine or osteopathy.
       L. *Primary Care Physician* means a Participating Physician who provides primary care services to Members (e.g., general or family practitioner, internist, pediatrician, or such other physician specialty as may be designated by the HMO). The Primary Care Physician is responsible for referrals of Members to Referral Physicians, other Participating Providers, and if necessary non-Participating Providers. Each Member shall select or have selected on his or her behalf a Primary Care Physician.

[Some HMOs allow for an OB/GYN to be designated as the primary care physician for all female enrollees or for pregnant members.]

       M. *Referral Physician* means a Participating Physician who is responsible for providing certain medical referral physician services upon referral by a Primary Care Physician.

N. *Service Area* means those counties in _____ set forth in Attachment A and such other areas as may be designated by the HMO from time to time.

[Although there is a reference to "Attachment A" in this section, no attachment is provided with the sample contract in this chapter. Chapter Three offered an in-depth discussion of payment methodologies and reimbursement terms that would be set forth in a typical "Attachment A."]

O. *Subscriber* means an individual who has contracted, or on whose behalf a contract has been entered into, with the HMO for health care services.

PART III. OBLIGATIONS OF THE PRIMARY CARE PHYSICIAN

A. *Health Services* The Primary Care Physician shall have the primary responsibility for arranging and coordinating the overall health care of Members, including appropriate referral to Participating Physicians and Participating Providers, and for managing and coordinating the performance of administrative functions relating to the delivery of health services to Members in accordance with this Agreement. In the event that the Primary Care Physician shall provide the Member with non-Covered Services, the Primary Care Physician shall, prior to the provision of such non-Covered Services, inform the Member:

1. of the service(s) to be provided,
2. that the HMO will not pay for or be liable for said services, and
3. that the Member will be financially liable for such services.

[This prior notification requirement is often required by state law.]

For any health care services rendered to or authorized for Members by the Primary Care Physician for which the HMO's prior approval is required and such prior approval was not obtained, the Primary Care Physician agrees that in no event will the HMO assume financial responsibility for charges arising from such services, and payments made by the HMO for such services may be deducted by the HMO from payments otherwise due the Primary Care Physician.

[Physicians should be informed of the circumstances or conditions for which prior HMO approval is required.]

B. *Referrals* Except in Emergencies or when authorized by the HMO, the Primary Care Physician agrees to make referrals of Members only to Participating Providers, and only in accordance with HMO policies. The Primary

Care Physician will furnish such Participating Providers complete information on treatment procedures and diagnostic tests performed prior to such referral. Upon referral, the Primary Care Physician agrees to notify the HMO of referral. In the event that services required by a Member are not available from the Participating Providers, non-Participating Physicians or Providers may be utilized with the prior approval of the HMO. The HMO will periodically furnish the Primary Care Physician with a current listing of the HMO's Participating Referral Physicians and Participating Providers.

C. *Hospital Admissions* In cases where a Member requires a non-Emergency Hospital admission, the Primary Care Physician agrees to secure authorization for such admission in accordance with the HMO's procedures prior to the admission. In addition, the Primary Care Physician agrees to abide by the HMO's Hospital discharge policies and procedures for Members.

[The administrative procedures manual (addressed in Part IV.A.) should clearly set forth all the requirements for prior authorization and discharges.]

D. *Primary Care Physician's Members* The Primary Care Physician shall not refuse to accept a Member as a patient on the basis of health status or medical condition of such Member, except with the approval of the Medical Director. The Primary Care Physician agrees to initiate closure of his or her practice to additional Members only if his or her practice, as a whole, is to be closed to additional patients or if authorized by the HMO. The Primary Care Physician may declare that he or she does not wish to accept additional Members (excluding persons already in the Primary Care Physician's practice that enroll in the HMO as Members) by giving the HMO written notice of such intent thirty (30) days in advance of the effective date of such closure. The Primary Care Physician agrees to accept any HMO Members seeking his or her services during the thirty (30) day notice period. A request for authorization by the HMO shall not be unreasonably denied.

In addition, a physician who is a Participating Provider may request, in writing to the HMO, that coverage for a Member be transferred to another Participating Physician. The Participating Physician shall not seek without authorization by the HMO to have a Member transferred because of the amount of services required by the Member or because of the health status of the Member.

E. *Charges to Members* Primary Care Physician shall accept as payment in full, for services which he or she provides, the compensation specified in Attachment B. The Primary Care Physician agrees that in no event, including, but not limited to, nonpayment, HMO insolvency, or breach of this Agreement, shall the Physician bill, charge, collect a deposit from, seek compensation, remuneration or reimbursement from, or have any recourse against Subscriber, Member, or persons other than the HMO acting on a Member's behalf for services provided pursuant to this Agreement. This provision shall not prohibit collection of copayments on the HMO's behalf made in accordance with the terms of the Evidence of Coverage between the HMO and Subscriber Member. The Primary Care Physician further agrees that:

1. this provision shall survive the termination of this Agreement regardless of the cause giving rise to termination and shall be construed to be for the benefit of the HMO Member, and that
2. this provision supersedes any oral or written contrary agreement now existing or hereafter entered into between the Primary Care Physician and Member, or persons acting on their behalf.

[The state department of insurance and the federal Health Care Financing Administration require that the provider agree not to bill a member except for deductibles, copayment, and noncovered services. Because this requirement and the specific language is usually dictated by state law, there is rarely any negotiating of these provisions.]

F. *Records and Reports*
1. The Primary Care Physician shall submit to the HMO for each Member an HMO Encounter Form, which shall contain such statistical and descriptive medical and patient data as specified by the HMO. The Primary Care Physician shall maintain such records and provide such medical, financial, and administrative information to the HMO as may be necessary for compliance by the HMO with state and federal law.

Primary Care Physician will further provide to HMO and, if required, to authorized state and federal agencies such access to medical records of HMO Members as is needed to ensure the quality of care rendered to such Members. HMO shall have access at reasonable times, upon request, to the billing and medical records of the Primary Care Physician relating to the health care services provided Members, and to information on the cost of such services, and on copayments received by the Primary Care Physician from Members for Covered Services. Utilization and cost data relating to a Participating Physician may be distributed by the HMO to other Participating Physicians for HMO program management purposes.
2. The HMO shall also have the right to inspect, at reasonable times, the Primary Care Physician's facilities pursuant to the HMO's credentialing, peer review, and quality assurance program.

3. The Primary Care Physician shall maintain a complete medical record for each Member in accordance with the requirements established by the HMO. Medical records of Members will include the recording of services provided by the Primary Care Physician, specialists, Hospitals, and other reports from referral providers, discharge summaries, records of Emergency care received by the Member, and such other information as the HMO requires.

[The primary care physician serves as gatekeeper and coordinator of care for this HMO. To serve this function, the primary care physician needs information from referral providers. There must be a requirement in a contract with referral physicians that this information be provided to the applicable primary care physician.]

Medical records of Members shall be treated as confidential so as to comply with all federal and state laws and regulations regarding the confidentiality of patient records. The HMO shall warrant that it has obtained any and all Member releases with respect to its access to such records.

[The payor usually requires that the provider allow for access to or copies of medical and financial records to verify coverage and payment. If access to such is to be accomplished through an on-site inspection, the payor should be required to do so in a manner that does not interfere with the normal business operations of the provider. Similarly, the payor should be required to reimburse the provider for reasonable copying costs of any records. For example, stating a specific cost per page or pegging it to the Medicare copying rate may avoid any question about the costs in the future. Often, providers are required to provide information to the state or the federal government as may be necessary for the payor to comply with state and federal laws.

If the contract calls for the provider to release patient-specific information, it is important to consider the requirements of state laws regarding confidentiality and prior patient authorization. The provider should also seek indemnification by the payor for any improper release of patient information that the payor obtains from the provider. The managed care organization should be the party responsible for obtaining a patient's release to review those medical records. Generally, those releases are contained as part of the enrollee application. Within the contract, the payor should represent and warrant that it has obtained any and all necessary member consents.

If the payor has not detailed a release with respect to certain protected categories of medical records, such as HIV or mental health and substance abuse, it may be appropriate for the primary care physician to make a good-faith attempt to obtain a patient's release for those records. The primary care physician cannot, however, represent that he or she it will be able to obtain a patient's consent with respect to any records, and payment should not be denied if the primary care physician is unable to obtain a patient's consent to release those records to the payor for purposes of UR/QA review.]

In most situations, a Member consents to release of his or her records as part of the HMO application and may necessitate special releases. Some HMOs require the Physician to obtain Member releases. Additionally, the contract should specify who is responsible for the cost of copying records requested pursuant to its utilization review process.

G. *Provision of Services and Professional Requirements*

1. The Primary Care Physician shall make necessary and appropriate arrangements to ensure the availability of physician services to his or her Member patients on a twenty-four (24) hour per day, seven (7) day per week basis, including arrangements to ensure coverage of his or her Member patients after hours or when the Primary Care Physician is otherwise absent, consistent with the HMO's administrative requirements. The Primary Care Physician agrees that scheduling of appointments for Members shall be done in a timely manner. The Primary Care Physician will maintain weekly appointment hours that are sufficient and convenient to serve Members and will maintain at all times Emergency and on-call services. Covering arrangements shall be with another Physician who is also a Participating Provider or who has otherwise been approved in advance by the HMO. For services rendered by any covering Physician on behalf of Primary Care Physician, including Emergency Services, it shall be the Primary Care Physician's sole responsibility to make suitable arrangements with the covering Physician regarding the manner in which said Physician will be reimbursed or otherwise compensated, provided, however, that the Primary Care Physician shall assure that the covering Physician will not, under any circumstances, bill HMO or bill Member for Covered Services (except co-payments), and the Primary Care Physician hereby agrees to indemnify and hold harmless Members and the HMO against charges for Covered Services rendered by physicians who are covering on behalf of the Primary Care Physician.

2. Primary Care Physician agrees:

A. not to discriminate in the treatment of his or her patients or in the quality of services delivered to HMO's Members on the basis of race, sex, age, religion, place of residence, health status, disability, or source of payment, and
B. to observe, protect, and promote the rights of Members as patients.

[The primary care physician shall not seek to transfer a member from his or her practice based on the member's health status, without authorization by the HMO. The physician may not be able to transfer a member because of his or her medical condition but may be able to seek transfer of the member on the grounds of the member's consistent noncompliance with medical directives.]

3. The Primary Care Physician agrees that all duties performed hereunder shall be consistent with the proper practice of medicine, and that such duties shall be performed in accordance with the customary rules of ethics and conduct of the applicable state and professional licensure boards and agencies. The Primary Care Physician shall use his or her own independent judgment as to the proper course of cure or treatment of his or her patients without regard to any agreement, provision, or understanding with the Plan.

[The physician could still be held liable for negligence if he or she does not exercise his or her own professional judgment and instead attempts to rely on the plan's utilization review process if, for example, a certain course of treatment is not authorized.]

4. The Primary Care Physician agrees that to the extent he or she utilizes allied Health Professionals and other personnel for delivery of health care, he or she will inform the HMO of the functions performed by such personnel.

5. The Primary Care Physician shall be duly licensed to practice medicine in _____ and shall maintain good professional standing at all times. Evidence of such licensing shall be submitted to the HMO upon request. In addition, the Primary Care Physician must meet all qualifications and standards for membership on the medical staff of at least one of the Hospitals, if any, that have contracted with the HMO and shall be required to maintain staff membership and full admission privileges in accordance with the rules and regulations of such Hospital and be otherwise acceptable to such Hospital. Finally, the Primary Care Physician shall be a duly qualified provider under the Medicare program. The Physician agrees to give immediate notice to the HMO in the case of suspension or revocation, or initiation of any proceeding that could result in suspension or revocation, of his or her licensure, Hospital privileges, or Medicare qualification status or the filing of a malpractice action against the Primary Care Physician.

[Although some of these items, such as reporting any malpractice suit, may not affect HMO Members, they all go to the question of the doctor's continuing competency to be part of the HMO provider panel. If the HMO has a separate credentialing process, the criteria should be specifically set forth or contained in an exhibit or attachment.]

H. *Insurance* The Primary Care Physician, including individual Physicians providing services to Members under this Agreement if the Primary Care Physician is a legal entity, shall provide and maintain such policies of general and professional liability (malpractice) insurance as shall be necessary to insure the Primary Care Physician and his or her employees against any claim or claims for damages arising by reason of personal injuries or death occasioned, directly or indirectly, in connection with the performance of any service by the Primary Care Physician. The amounts and extent of such insurance coverage shall be subject to the approval of the HMO. The Primary Care Physician shall provide memorandum copies of such insurance coverage to the HMO upon request.

[The amount of insurance that is acceptable should be set forth in the administrative procedures manual (Part IV.A.) or elsewhere. An HMO may request to be named as additional insured on the physician's policy, though this is usually considered an onerous and unnecessary level of protection for an HMO.]

I. *Administration*
1. The Primary Care Physician agrees to cooperate and participate in such review and service programs as may be established by the HMO, including utilization and quality assurance programs, credentialing, sanctioning, external audit systems, administrative procedures, and Member and Physician grievance procedures. The Primary Care Physician shall comply with all determinations rendered through the above programs.

[The administrative procedures manual (Part IV.A.) should spell out the details of all such programs and procedures, including an appeals process for UR.]

2. The Primary Care Physician agrees that the HMO may use his or her name, address, phone number, picture, type of practice, applicable practice restrictions, and an indication of the Primary Care Physician's willingness to accept additional Members in the HMO's roster of physician participants and other HMO materials. The Primary Care Physician shall not refer to the HMO in any publicity, advertisements, notices, or promotional material or in any announcement to the Members without prior review and written approval of the HMO.
3. The Primary Care Physician agrees to provide to the HMO information for the collection and coordination of benefits when a Member holds other coverage that is deemed primary for the provision of services to said Member and to abide by the HMO coordination-of-benefits and duplicate-coverage policies. This shall include, but not be limited to, permitting the HMO to bill and process forms for any third-party payor on the Primary Care Physician's behalf for Covered Services and to retain any sums received. In addition, the Primary Care Physician shall cooperate in and abide by the HMO subrogation policies and procedures.

[The primary care physician should share in any recovery of medical costs by the HMO via coordination of benefits. It is especially important to state this requirement explicitly in cases in which the physician is reimbursed on a capitation basis.]

4. The Primary Care Physician agrees to maintain the confidentiality of all information related to fees, charges, expenses, and utilization derived from, through, or provided by the HMO.

5. The Primary Care Physician warrants and represents that all information and statements given to the HMO in applying for or maintaining his or her HMO Primary Care Physician Agreement are true, accurate, and complete. The HMO Physician application shall be incorporated by reference into this Agreement. Any inaccurate or incomplete information or misrepresentation of information provided by the Primary Care Physician may result in the immediate termination of the Agreement by the HMO.

6. The Primary Care Physician shall cooperate with the HMO in complying with applicable laws relating to the HMO.

PART IV. OBLIGATIONS OF THE HMO

A. *Administrative Procedures* The HMO shall make available to the Primary Care Physician a manual of administrative procedures (including any changes thereto) in the areas of recordkeeping, reporting, and other administrative duties of the Primary Care Physician under this Agreement. The Primary Care Physician agrees to abide by such administrative procedures.

[Most HMOs have administrative procedure manuals that cover the details of claims processing, utilization review, quality assurance, etc. These manuals should always be reviewed as an important part of the contract and should only be amended on, for example, ninety (90) days' prior notice to guard against significant and unacceptable modifications to any process.]

B. *Compensation* For all Medically Necessary Covered Services provided to Members by the Primary Care Physician, the HMO shall pay to the Primary Care Physician the compensation set forth in Attachment B.

[Attachment B in the sample contract of this chapter sets forth alternative language for an HMO that pays its primary care physicians on either a fee-for-service or a capitated basis. The purpose of the risk-sharing incentive compensation arrangement set forth in Attachment B is to monitor utilization; control costs of health services, including hospitalization; and achieve utilization goals while maintaining quality of care.]

Itemized statements on HMO Encounter Forms, or approved equivalent, for all Covered Services rendered by the Primary Care Physician must be submitted to the HMO within ninety (90) days of the date the service was rendered in order to be compensated by the HMO.

C. *Processing of Claims* The HMO agrees to process Primary Care Physician claims for Covered Services rendered to Members. The HMO will make payment within thirty (30) days from the date the claim is received. Where a claim requires additional documentation, the HMO will make payment within thirty (30) days from date of receipt of sufficient documentation to approve the claim. If the HMO fails to pay the Physician within thirty (30) days, interest shall accrue at the rate of 12 percent per annum retroactive to the date of service.

[This paragraph allows the HMO to delay payment to the physician while waiting for sufficient documentation. What constitutes a "clean" or complete claim should be clearly set forth in the administrative procedures manual.]

D. *Eligibility Report* The HMO shall provide the Primary Care Physician with a monthly listing of eligible Members who have selected or have been assigned to the Primary Care Physician.

[The HMO should also have a mechanism for telephone verification of eligibility.]

E. *Reports* The HMO will provide the Primary Care Physician with periodic statements with respect to the compensation set forth in Attachment B and with utilization reports in accordance with the HMO's administrative procedures. The Primary Care Physician agrees to maintain the confidentiality of the information presented in such reports.

[To enable the physician to review utilization information and, if appropriate, adjust behavior, detailed reports should be provided by the HMO to the physician at least quarterly and preferably monthly.]

PART V. MISCELLANEOUS

A. *Modification of This Agreement* This Agreement may be amended or modified in writing as mutually agreed upon by the parties. In addition, the HMO may modify any provision of this Agreement upon thirty (30) days' prior written notice to the Primary Care Physician. The Primary Care Physician shall be deemed to have accepted the HMO's modification if the Primary Care Physician fails to object to such modification, in writing, within the thirty (30) day notice period. If the Physician does so object, this Agreement shall remain in full force and effect, absent said modification, for the remainder of the term of the Agreement.

[This is a common provision and useful in simplifying the administrative work associated with amending the agreement. Needless to say, it is important for the HMO to explain clearly to the primary care physician the nature of the amendment.]

B. *Interpretation* This Agreement shall be governed in all respects by the laws of the State of _____. The invalidity or unenforceability of any terms or conditions hereof shall in no way affect the validity or enforceability of any other terms or provisions. The waiver by either party of a breach or violation of any provision of this Agreement shall not operate as or be construed to be a waiver of any subsequent breach thereof.

C. *Assignment* Neither party may assign this Agreement without the prior consent of the other party.

D. *Notice* Any notice required to be given pursuant to the terms and provisions hereof shall be sent by certified mail, return receipt requested, postage prepaid, to the HMO or to the Primary Care Physician at the respective addresses indicated herein. Notice shall be deemed to be effective when mailed, but notice of change of address shall be effective upon receipt.

E. *Relationship of Parties* None of the provisions of this Agreement is intended to create nor shall be deemed or construed to create any relationship between the parties hereto other than that of independent entities contracting with each other hereunder solely for the purpose of effecting the provisions of this Agreement. Neither of the parties hereto, nor any of their respective employees, shall be construed to be the agent, employer, employee, or representative of the other, nor will either party have an express or implied right of authority to assume or create any obligation or responsibility on behalf of or in the name of the other party.

F. *Gender* The use of any gender herein shall be deemed to include the other gender where applicable.

G. *Legal Entity* If the Primary Care Physician is a legal entity, an application for each Physician who is a member of such entity must be submitted to and accepted by the HMO before such Physician may serve as a Primary Care Physician under this Agreement.

H. *Term and Termination* The term of this Agreement shall be for three (3) years from the effective date set forth on the signature page. This Agreement may be terminated by either party at any time without cause by prior written notice given at least sixty (60) days in advance of the effective date of such termination. This Agreement may also be terminated by the HMO effective immediately upon written notice if the Primary Care Physician's (or if a legal entity, any of the entity's physicians') medical license, Medicare qualification, or Hospital privileges are suspended, limited, restricted, or revoked, or if the Primary

Care Physician violates Subsections (E), (G), or (H) herein. Upon termination, the rights of each party hereunder shall terminate, provided, however, that such action shall not release the Primary Care Physician or HMO from their obligations with respect to:

1. payments accrued to the Primary Care Physician prior to termination;
2. the Primary Care Physician's agreement not to seek compensation from Members for Covered Services provided prior to termination; and
3. completion of treatment of Members then receiving care until continuation of the Member's care can be arranged by the HMO.

In the event of termination, no distribution of any money accruing to the Primary Care Physician under the provisions of Attachment B shall be made until the regularly scheduled date for such distributions. Upon termination, the HMO is empowered and authorized to notify Members and prospective Members, other Primary Care Physicians, and other persons or entities whom it deems to have an interest herein of such termination, through such means as it may choose.

[The primary care physician may want to review the form of a letter notifying members of a physician's termination from the HMO panel.]

In the event of notice of termination, the HMO may notify Members of such fact and assign Members to or require Members to select another Primary Care Physician prior to the effective date of termination. In any event, the HMO shall continue to compensate the Primary Care Physician until the effective date of termination as provided herein for those Members who, because of health reasons, cannot be assigned or make such selection during the notice of termination period and as provided by the HMO's Medical Director. Payment for any services provided by Physician to the Member after the termination of this Agreement shall be at Physician's charges.

IN WITNESS WHEREOF, the foregoing Agreement between _____ _____ and Primary Care Physician is entered into by and between the undersigned parties, to be effective this _____ day of _____, 19___.

Primary Care Physician _____

_____   By: _____

(Name of individual physician or of
group practice—please print)

_____   _____
(Mailing address)   (Date)

_____
(City, state, zip)

_____
(Telephone number)

_____
(Taxpayer identification number)

_____
(DEA number)

_____
(Signature)

_____
(Name and title if signing as authorized representative of group practice)

_____
(Date)

Attachment B
Compensation Schedule
Primary Care Physician Agreement

*[This attachment describes one form of fee-for-service-with-withhold methodology for primary
care physician payment. Chapter Three offered in-depth discussion of various methodologies and
payment terms.]*

I. SERVICES RENDERED BY PHYSICIANS

For Covered Services provided by the Primary Care Physician in accordance
with the terms of this Agreement, HMO shall pay the Primary Care Physician
his or her Reimbursement Allowance, less any applicable copayment for which
the Member is responsible under the applicable Evidence of Coverage and less
the Withhold Amount, as described below. "Reimbursement Allowance" shall
mean the lower of (1) the usual and customary fee charged by the Primary
Care Physician for the Covered Service, or (2) the maximum amount allowed
under the fee limits established by the HMO.

II. WITHHOLDS FROM REIMBURSEMENT ALLOWANCE

The HMO shall withhold from each payment to the Primary Care Physician
a percentage of the Reimbursement Allowance ("Withhold Amount") and
shall allocate an amount equal to such withhold to an HMO Risk Fund. The
HMO shall have the right, in its sole discretion, to modify the percentage withheld from the Primary Care Physician if, in its judgment, the financial condition, operations, or commitments of the HMO or its expenses for particular
health services or for services by any particular Participating Providers warrant
such modification.

III. WITHHOLD AMOUNT DISTRIBUTIONS

The HMO may, at its sole discretion, from time to time distribute to the
Primary Care Physician Withhold Amounts retained by HMO from payments to the Primary Care Physician, plus such additional amounts, if any,
that the HMO may deem appropriate as a financial incentive to the provision
of cost-effective health care services. The HMO may, from time to time, com-
mit or expend Withhold Amounts, in whole or in part, to ensure the financial
stability of or commitments of the HMO or health care plans or payors with
or for which the HMO has an agreement to arrange for the provision of
health care services, or to satisfy budgetary or financial objectives established
by the HMO.

Subject to the HMO's peer review procedures and policies, a Primary
Care Physician may be excluded from any distribution if he or she does not

qualify for such distribution, i.e., if he or she has exceeded HMO utilization standards or criteria. No Primary Care Physician shall have any entitlement to any funds in the HMO Risk Fund.

IV. ACCOUNTING

The Primary Care Physician shall be entitled to an accounting of Withhold Amounts from payments to him or her upon written request to the HMO.

Attachment B (Alternate)
Capitation Payment
Primary Care Physician Agreement

[This attachment describes a form of capitation primary care physician payment methodology. Chapter Three offered in-depth discussion of various methodologies and payment terms.]

COMPENSATION
I. CAPITATION ALLOCATION
The total monthly amounts paid to the Primary Care Physician will be determined as follows:

For each Member selecting the Primary Care Physician ("selecting" also includes Members assigned to a Primary Care Physician), 90 percent of the monthly Primary Care Service capitation set forth below for Primary Care Services shall be paid by the HMO to the Primary Care Physician by the 5th day of the following month. The capitation shall be set according to the particular benefit plan in which each Member is enrolled. Where the capitation is not currently adjusted for age and/or sex, the HMO reserves the right to make such age and/or sex adjustment to the capitation rates upon thirty (30) days' notice.

The HMO shall allocate the remaining 10 percent of the monthly capitation payments to a Risk Reserve Fund, which fund is subject to the further provisions of this Attachment. The capitation payments to the Primary Care Physician for Primary Care Services, subject to the above withhold, are as follows:

Coverage Plans

Age and Sex	Commercial Plan A Capitation Payment	Commercial Plan B Capitation Payment	Commercial Plan C Capitation Payment
24 months, M or F	$_____	$_____	$_____
2–4 years, M or F	$_____	$_____	$_____
5–19 years, F	$_____	$_____	$_____
5–19 years, M	$_____	$_____	$_____
20–39 years, F	$_____	$_____	$_____
20–39 years, M	$_____	$_____	$_____
40–49 years, F	$_____	$_____	$_____
40–49 years, M	$_____	$_____	$_____
50–59 years, F	$_____	$_____	$_____
50–59 years, M	$_____	$_____	$_____
>60 years, F	$_____	$_____	$_____
>60 years, M	$_____	$_____	$_____

The Primary Care Physician is financially liable for all Primary Care Services rendered to Members under the above capitation. If the Primary Care Physician fails to do so, the HMO may pay for such services on behalf of the Primary Care Physician and deduct such payments from any sums otherwise due the Primary Care Physician by the HMO.

CHAPTER SEVEN

MANAGED CARE OPERATIONS

What's the next step? Organizing managed care operations. Recommendations for delineating key roles and responsibilities and using information systems to support managed care operations are provided in this chapter.

Managed care operations are often highly fragmented in a hospital or large physician organization. A variety of functional departments have to design specific policies and procedures to address issues unique to managed care. Exhibit 7.1 provides an overview of key responsibilities by functional department. In reality, to "manage managed care," the provider needs even more information and data spanning a variety of functional areas.

A managed care contract manual should be developed and routinely maintained to keep a concise and easily accessible record of key contracts and contract terms. Components of the contract manual might be:

- Managed care strategy statement (derived during the planning phase)
- Copies of contracts (perhaps with limited dissemination of information to select individuals)
- Copies of plan ID cards and telephone numbers
- Calendar of renewal dates, including termination notice requirements and effective dates)
- List of contact people and telephone numbers

EXHIBIT 7.1. FUNCTIONAL REQUIREMENTS FOR MANAGED CARE.

Department	Things to Do
Administrative management	Develop the managed care strategy. Develop an appropriate organizational structure for assignment of managed care responsibility, coordination of external support functions (e.g., consulting, legal, actuarial, claims processing), interaction with existing and potential managed care subsidiaries, and subcontracting with ancillary providers. Identify perceived strengths of the organization. Design appropriate reports to document perceived strengths. Identify weaknesses of the organization. Work with appropriate service delivery departments to develop mechanisms to correct weaknesses and performance standards and a monitoring methodology to measure improvements in problem areas. Gather input from other departments regarding contractual concerns or limitations, and incorporate these into the negotiating strategy. Develop the negotiating strategy.
Planning	Subscribe to pertinent managed care publications. Collect and disseminate trend data in managed care and in area employment. Develop database of state HMO filings and update quarterly or annually.
Marketing and public relations	Develop guidelines for use of provider's name in other entities' advertising and promotional copy. Design database of employer market data. Develop patient satisfaction surveys. Package wellness programs to enhance managed care image.
Finance	Obtain and maintain copies of all managed care contracts (file in the contract manual). Compile lists of participating physicians by existing managed care program. Accumulate assumptions used to develop financial terms under existing managed care contracts. Develop worksheets for purpose of preparing a financial analysis of new and renewal contractual arrangements. Design reports that provide data by employer group, by payor, and by benefit plan. Design cost accounting variance reporting formats.
Outpatient registration	Revise registration forms and procedures to include new data fields, as required. Document eligibility verification and authorization procedures in quick reference format.

	Identify contractual documentation burdens for consideration in future contract negotiations. Develop procedures for collecting patient copayments and deductibles.
Billing and collection	Identify and document specific billing requirements by payor. Identify system constraints and develop methods to remedy them. Identify late-payment penalties by payor, and incorporate in collection process.
Patient care	Establish cost accounting standards by activity performed. Establish performance standards in conjunction with administrative management to correct operational deficiencies. Modify forms to collect statistical data on key performance measures. Identify key service deficiencies for enhancements in level or type of service.
Emergency room	Develop procedures for collecting patient copayments and deductibles. Develop procedures for contacting primary care physicians as appropriate. Develop procedures for eligibility and benefit verification. Document eligibility verification and authorization procedures in quick reference format. Identify contractual documentation burdens for consideration in future contract negotiations.
Utilization review	Design reports of utilization (by actual procedural-level usage) by physician. Document current UR procedures by payor. Define functional and liability limitations on UR activities to be performed by provider staff. Develop procedures to coordinate with billing payment limitations. Design daily monitoring logs for utilization controls. Identify communication mechanism for QA/UR feedback.
Social services	Develop integrated discharge planning process in conjunction with UR and OP service departments.
Quality assurance and infection control	Design system for accumulation of morbidity, mortality, and infection statistics for selected tertiary-level diagnoses and by physician by specialty.
Information systems	Add needed fields and linkages to database (e.g., employer in addition to third-party payor). Code reports designed by other functional areas

- Distribution list for manual to keep track of all individuals involved in the managed care process
- Worksheet that identifies key contract information
- Contract review checklist

Routine financial reporting requirements also have to be established to monitor a provider's financial performance under managed care contracts. Here are examples of the key financial performance measures:

Monthly Reporting Requirements

1. For all risk arrangements
   A. Net revenues compared to actual variable cost (based on procedure-level cost accounting)
   B. Gross and net revenue by payor
   C. Contribution margin by payor (based on procedure-level cost accounting)
   D. Average age of receivables by payor
   E. Volume by type of service
2. For capitation contracts
   A. Per member per month cost analysis
      - Fee for service equivalents
      - Actual variable cost based on procedure-level costing
   B. Withhold or risk-pool summary
3. For percentage of premium arrangements
   A. Premium yield compared to budget PMPM
   B. Premium yield by benefit plan
   C. Premium yield by employer group

Annual Reporting Requirements

1. Enrollment projections by plan
   A. By key employer group
   B. By zip code
2. Utilization projections by plan by service
3. Procedural costing by service
4. Settlement of risk pools
5. Line-of-business financial statements

As providers move into more integrated systems (Figure 7.1), the management information system needs vary, as Figure 7.2 shows. Concurrently, the role of information technology must match the demands generated at each stage.

As market characteristics evolve, and managed care demands increase, a provider must add many additional modules to its information system capabilities.

Health care professionals often incorrectly assume that the information system capabilities that were adequate for indemnity-driven reimbursement (contract management) are applicable for managed care contracting and management. Figure 7.3 displays the high-level functionality that traditionally was associated with contract management. In thinking about a provider's managed care information needs, one must further "drill down" or refine an information system's functionality. Some of the comparative functional needs are presented in Figure 7.4.

In regard to managed care software, a provider must anticipate how its particular market is evolving as it decides the degree of managed care information capabilities it may need. A vendor continuum is displayed in Figure 7.5. The

FIGURE 7.1. INTEGRATED DELIVERY SYSTEM STAGES.

Stages of Transition
- There are three basic stages of transition into a fully integrated health care delivery system
- Information system needs vary based on the integrated delivery system's current stage, and the pace at which they are willing and able to move toward full integration.

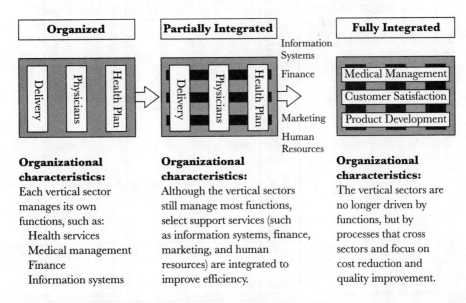

Organizational characteristics:
Each vertical sector manages its own functions, such as:
   Health services
   Medical management
   Finance
   Information systems

Organizational characteristics:
Although the vertical sectors still manage most functions, select support services (such as information systems, finance, marketing, and human resources) are integrated to improve efficiency.

Organizational characteristics:
The vertical sectors are no longer driven by functions, but by processes that cross sectors and focus on cost reduction and quality improvement.

FIGURE 7.2. INFORMATION TECHNOLOGY STAGES ON THE WAY.

In a parallel vein, the role of information technology within the evolving integrated health care system must match the demands generated at each stage . . . . .

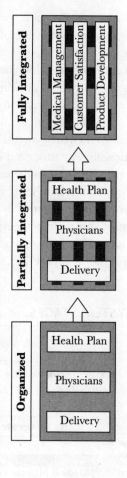

Information Technology Roles	Organizational Stage		
	Organized	Partially Integrated	Fully Integrated
Process automation	Increase clerical and clinical efficiency Increase administrative efficiency	Customer and member access focus Integration authorization and referral	Physician focus on clinical process management Process management by exception
Integration	Campus or care site Basic medical utilization data Physician to hospital	Enterprise connectivity and integration Episode clinical data repository and data access	External community connectivity Lifetime clinical data
Measurement and management of outcomes	Initial support for episode management (care maps and protocols) Support manual accumulation of outcomes data	Member service value Enterprisewide service and performance data Service-line value analysis	Health status Embedded clinical process management

FIGURE 7.3. CONTRACT MANAGEMENT SYSTEMS: HIGH-LEVEL FUNCTIONALITY.

Contract Negotiation	Preadmission Screening	Concurrent Screening, Utilization Review, Quality Monitoring	Billing and Accounts Receivable	Tracking Contract Performance
• Resource utilization • Patient clinical and demographic characteristics • Forecasting/modeling – Stop-loss clauses – Trim factors – Effect of cost, revenue, or activity changes on total revenues, products, service lines • Variable and fixed costs • Flexible budgeting by contract – Revenue – Cost – Utilization	• Eligibility verification • Contract requirements – Admission criteria – Contract terms – Effective dates • Calculation of expected reimbursement	• Utilization review – Authorization of continued stay • Resource utilization – Control costs – Assure quality of care • Decision support – Integration of clinical and financial data with payor criteria • Discharge planning – Coverage for continuing care treatment	• Expected reimbursement for payors • Contractual allowance at time of billing • Explanatory billing invoices – Expected reimbursement by contract • Comparison reporting – Actual versus expected payment • Automatic posting of contractual allowances – General ledger – Patient accounting	• Comparison reporting of actual usage versus contract budgets – Utilization – Cost – Revenue – Margins • Resource utilization history – Distribution of cost – Specific outliers – Clinical indicators

associated software and implementation costs vary as much as the array of possible vendors. The total costs vary from a minimum of $50,000 to several million dollars at the high end.

As one of our clients once put it: "We discuss at length the type and investment in information systems. To me, I draw the following analogy: if you don't have your own data source, it is tantamount to playing poker with a gambler who insists on using his own deck of cards."

FIGURE 7.4. CONTRACT MANAGEMENT SYSTEMS: CONTRACT MANAGEMENT VERSUS MANAGED CARE.

Contract Management vs. Managed Care	
• Model payor contracts • Alert for expiring contracts • Track patients when admitted to or discharged from hospital • Maintain physician group contract information • Maintain information on authorization requirements • Verify patient benefit information • Price bills at contract rates • Generate an explanation of reimbursement (EOR)	• Store vendor contracts for claims administration • Maintain enrollment history of all members • Monitor benefit utilization to track out-of-pocket maximums, copays, and benefit limitations • Track specialist referrals • Provide utilization review and case management functions • Maintain terms of provider contracts • Adjudicate claim according to eligibility, benefits, authorizations, and provider contract • Generate a check and EOB

FIGURE 7.5. MANAGED CARE SOFTWARE.

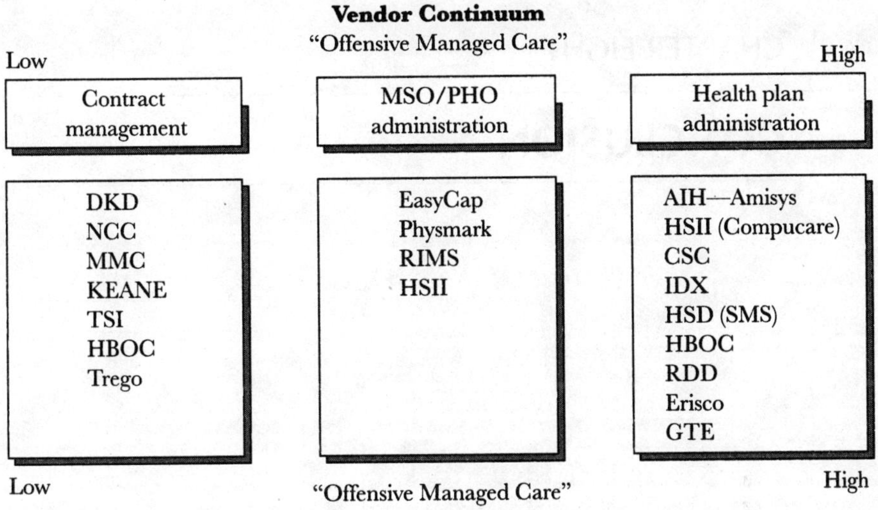

Vendor Continuum
"Offensive Managed Care"

Low   High

Contract management	MSO/PHO administration	Health plan administration
DKD NCC MMC KEANE TSI HBOC Trego	EasyCap Physmark RIMS HSII	AIH—Amisys HSII (Compucare) CSC IDX HSD (SMS) HBOC RDD Erisco GTE

Low   "Offensive Managed Care"   High

CHAPTER EIGHT

CONCLUSION

Managed care contracting is becoming increasingly complex. Each provider needs to assess the market and competitive environment in which it operates, and because those market forces are shifting constantly this becomes an ongoing evaluation. A hospital that had substantial leverage yesterday may lose competitive advantage tomorrow to an institution that is substantially integrating with its physicians and other providers. A large managed care organization that has had a significant number of members may now be experiencing financial problems and be under the scrutiny of the state department of insurance or corporations. A medical group with clout in the community may lose a leading physician. Moreover, since many managed care contracts are for specific terms of one, two, or three years, the parties may be forced to review the process and renegotiate the terms of the agreement every few years.

For providers embarking on managed care contracting or refining their approach, an appropriate strategy and organized methodology, as described in this book, will serve them well. These efforts, however, should not be a one-time event for providers. Once providers enter into a contract with a plan, they should continuously review competitive factors, operational strengths and weaknesses (of both the payor and internally of the provider), financial performance, MIS capability, medical management, claims processing, and administrative responsiveness. The checklists and criteria described for initial contracting activities should become part of a continual evaluation process.

Similarly, the provider's expectations with respect to evaluating an initial proposal should be compared with actual experience. Have the objectives of the provider been accomplished? Have financial expectations been achieved? Where are the strengths in the relationship with the plan? Where are the weaknesses? Is the provider collecting and reviewing the proper information to assess the agreement? Is the right team evaluating the relationship?

As with the initial considerations, the ongoing review process should ultimately lead to modifications in the written agreement. The agreement will be modified, and the providers should continue to monitor and evaluate the relationship in accordance with the guidelines described in earlier chapters for further amendments to the contract likely to arise in the future.

INDEX

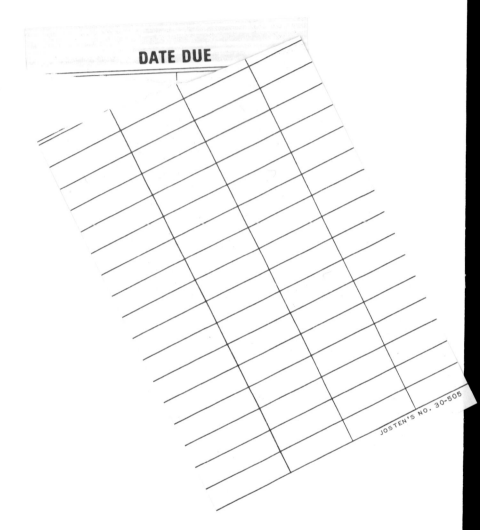